About this book

The Male Factor explores the influence of sperm health on fertility outcomes, an area that has long been underestimated and oversimplified in reproductive care. Even though male factors contribute to at least 50% of infertility cases, the burden of investigation and treatment has traditionally fallen on those assigned female at birth. They are often the ones scheduling appointments, undergoing blood tests, and facing expensive and invasive procedures, while male factor fertility and sperm health assessment are frequently delayed, incomplete, or overlooked.

Written by Raul Pastrana, an experienced naturopath who has supported hundreds of couples, this book is grounded in clinical experience and evidence-based research. It examines the wide range of factors that influence male fertility, including hormonal, anatomical, metabolic, genetic, environmental, and lifestyle contributors, and explains how these directly impact sperm health and reproductive outcomes.

A key theme of the book is the gap between being told that sperm results are "normal" and what truly represents healthy, optimised sperm. Raul draws on his clinical expertise and extensive research to challenge outdated sperm reference ranges and introduce more meaningful benchmarks that better reflect sperm quality and reproductive potential.

This book serves as a practical guide for couples who want to share responsibility in their fertility journey by actively addressing and improving sperm health. It is written for those trying to conceive naturally, as well as for couples undergoing IVF who wish to optimise their chances of success.

Rather than focusing on diagnosis alone, *The Male Factor* encourages a more human and realistic approach to fertility care, one that recognises shared responsibility, early investigation, and treatment tailored to the individual. By changing how male fertility is understood and addressed, this book aims to support better decision-making, improve treatment outcomes, and ultimately increase the chances of a successful pregnancy and live birth.

About the Author: Raul Pastrana (he/him) BHSc (Nat)

Raul is a degree-qualified naturopath and recognized expert in fertility and reproductive health, with a strong focus on male fertility. He is LGBTQIA+ friendly and passionate about breaking down complex health topics into practical insights for a broad audience.

With expertise spanning male and female fertility, gut health, menopause, and weight management, Raul combines evidence-based nutrition, herbal medicine, and lifestyle strategies to help individuals and couples optimize their health and reproductive outcomes.

Raul is particularly known for his deep understanding of lifestyle's impact on fertility, drawing on his experience as a personal trainer to help people integrate meaningful change into daily life. He brings a fresh, engaging perspective to discussions on health, wellness, and fertility, making him a sought-after voice for podcasts, magazine features, and expert commentary.

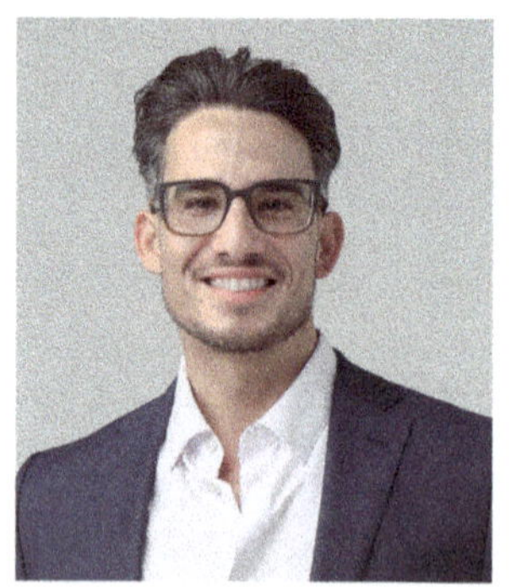

Contact

Website: www.rhreproductivehealth.com

Email: raul@rhreproductivehealth.com

Instagram: @raulpastrana_hormonalhealth

Medical Disclaimer

The information provided in *The Male Factor* is intended for educational and informational purposes only. It is not medical advice, nor is it intended to replace consultation, diagnosis, or treatment from a qualified healthcare professional.

While every effort has been made to ensure the accuracy and reliability of the information presented, fertility, hormonal health, and medical conditions are complex and individual. What is appropriate for one person may not be appropriate for another.

Readers are strongly encouraged to consult their doctor, specialist, or qualified healthcare provider before making any changes to their diet, supplementation, lifestyle, medications, or treatment plan. This is particularly important if you have an existing medical condition, are taking prescribed medications, are undergoing fertility treatment (including IVF), or are preparing for conception.

Copyright Notice

A note on language

For the purpose of this book, the term male is used to refer to individuals assigned male at birth (AMAB), and female to those assigned female at birth (AFAB). We acknowledge that gender identity and expression are diverse and may not align with these biological classifications. My intention is to discuss reproductive health using terminology relevant to anatomy and physiology, while remaining respectful and inclusive of all gender identities.

Index

Chapter 1

Why this book?

If you are holding this book, chances are you've felt the weight of fertility challenges. Maybe in your own body, maybe watching your partner carry almost all the responsibility. For too long, males have been left out of the conversation. Fertility has been treated as a female's issue, when in reality it is half sperm and half egg. Half responsibility, half opportunity. Yet when couples struggle to conceive, it is usually females who are tested, medicated, and guided through endless protocols, while males are often told little more than "your sperm is fine" or "just be healthy." This is not only unfair, but also inaccurate. Research shows that up to half of all infertility cases involve male factors. And even when conception happens, sperm health still plays a crucial role in pregnancy and offspring health outcomes.

This book exists because that narrative needs to change. Those creating the sperm deserve clear, practical guidance on how their everyday choices affect fertility, miscarriage risk, pregnancy, and their future child's health. Too many males are never given this information, and too many females are left to carry the responsibility alone. I aim to make the science simple, to give you the tools you can actually use, and to reframe fertility as a shared journey. When both members of the couple step up and do their part, the chances of success improve, the emotional load is shared more fairly, and it is possible to move forward as a stronger team.

So, let me introduce myself. My name is Raul Pastrana, and I am a naturopathic practitioner working in reproductive health. I am based in Melbourne, Australia, and I work with patients both locally and internationally via telehealth, alongside my colleagues at RH Reproductive Health.

A large part of my work is supporting individuals and couples facing fertility challenges. Often, by the time I see a couple for the first time, they have already been trying for one, two, sometimes even three years without success. My role is to review what has been done so far, identify what may have been overlooked, and uncover the barriers standing in the way of conception.

Over the years, I've noticed a pattern that is impossible to ignore. Females' partners usually arrive with folders of blood tests, scans, supplements, and detailed treatment histories. On the other hand, male patients often arrive with little or nothing. Sometimes, just a semen analysis conducted via a poor-quality lab with unreliable results, and rarely with a proper assessment or plan for improving sperm health. I've seen couples being pushed toward invasive, stressful, and very expensive fertility treatments, when in some cases, the issue could have been addressed much more simply if the male factor had been properly investigated and supported. This gap in care is not only frustrating but also unfair. And it is exactly why this book needed to be written.

<u>Why me? Why am I the one writing this book about sperm health?</u>

I was born and raised in Madrid, Spain, in a family where health was always a priority. My mother ensured that my sister and I grew up with good food, strong values, and an understanding that taking care of ourselves is one of life's most important assets. Those early lessons shaped the way I see health today. Not a choice, but as the foundation for everything else.

When I moved to Australia in 2014, I brought those values with me. Very soon, I found myself working as a personal trainer, something that felt like a natural step, since I had been going to the gym for most of my adult life and genuinely enjoyed it. Fitness wasn't just a job; it was part of who I was.

As a PT, I worked with males who wanted to improve their performance, energy, and confidence. One of the things I noticed quickly was that the gym does far more than build muscle; it builds confidence. When a person sees themselves getting stronger, lifting weights they couldn't move a few weeks earlier, it changes the way they carry themselves outside the gym, too. If you haven't tried it, I encourage you to give it a go. Confidence isn't just about appearance; it's about what you prove to yourself when you show up consistently and see progress.

Over time, I also saw the deeper patterns: how much hormones, lifestyle, and daily habits could influence not only physical results but also mood, motivation, and overall wellbeing. Those years gave me valuable insight into the way the male bodies respond to stress, nutrition, training, and recovery. These were all factors which later became central to my work in fertility and reproductive health.

Following this, I decided to dive deeper and study naturopathy, specialising in fertility and hormonal health, which allowed me to connect the dots. The same males who struggled with energy or recovery in the gym often faced fertility challenges in the clinic. By combining my background in fitness with my clinical practice, I now assist couples in understanding what's really going on, especially when it comes to the often-overlooked sperm factor.

This mix of personal origins, years of experience with male performance, and a clinical focus on fertility is what makes me uniquely positioned to write this book. I understand both the science and the practical, everyday steps that males can take. My goal is simple: to make sperm health approachable, to share strategies that work, and to give you the clarity and confidence to finally do your part.

Is this book for you?

This book is for those who want to do their part in the fertility journey. Whether or not you've ever had a semen analysis, whether your results were normal, excellent, or far from ideal, there is always something you can do to support your partner and improve outcomes. Fertility isn't just about sperm counts and lab reports; it's about responsibility, teamwork, and making practical changes that give both you and your partner the best possible chance of success.

Preconception care for males is often overlooked, but it is a huge factor affecting your outcomes. Maybe your sperm health has never been checked. Maybe your results looked fine, but you want to be proactive and do everything possible to share the responsibility with your partner.

Or maybe you've already been told that your sperm health isn't ideal, and you want to know how it can be improved. In every case, the steps in this book are relevant, realistic, and designed to make a measurable difference in your sperm health.

If you've had a semen analysis but the results weren't ideal, don't lose hope. Sperm are produced in a cycle called *spermatogenesis*, which takes around seventy-two to seventy-four days. That means you can start creating healthier sperm in less than three months if you begin making changes now. No shortcuts, no gimmicks, just evidence-based steps that work.

Even if natural conception isn't possible and you're moving towards assisted reproductive technologies (ART) like in vitro fertilisation (IVF) or intracytoplasmic sperm injection (ICSI), sperm quality still matters. Improving it can increase your chances of success, reduce the number of treatment rounds, lower costs, and ease the emotional strain for both you and your partner.

And here's the good news: the same actions that improve sperm also enhance overall health. More energy. Better sleep. Sharper focus. Stronger erections. Better cardiovascular fitness. All of these are positive side effects of taking care of yourself.

That's why I wrote this book. I've seen too many females carry this burden alone, booking appointments, getting tests, changing diets, and feeling the weight of responsibility. Meanwhile, their partners are often left unsure of what role they can play. That imbalance needs to change.

If you're holding this book, it's because you already care. You want to support your partner, improve your chances of a healthy pregnancy, and give your future child the strongest start possible.

So why not dedicate three months of your life to giving your future family the best possible start? Fertility is a shared responsibility. It's time for you to step up and say,

"I'm 50 percent of this. I won't let my partner carry it alone. I'm ready to do my part."

Let's do it together. I'll help you *do your part* in this fertility journey.

This book will show you how. You'll learn what affects sperm health, what to avoid, and the daily steps you can take to improve both the quality and quantity of your sperm. The information here is clear, practical, and ready for you to use.

Raul Pastrana

Chapter 2

Introduction to male fertility

<u>Importance of male fertility in conception</u>

Sperm plays a vital role in the creation of life, contributing half of the genetic material needed to form a viable embryo. Despite the common misconception that fertility issues primarily concern women, research shows that sperm-related factors are either wholly or partially responsible for half of all infertility cases.

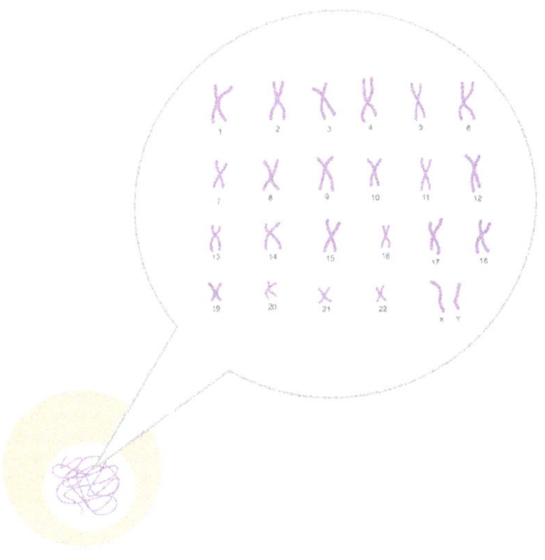

Given these statistics, investing the time and money through a complete semen analysis is more than worthwhile. It gives you a clear picture of your current fertility baseline and helps to set realistic goals for improvement.

A standard semen analysis evaluates three key parameters:

- ☐ Count: how many sperm are present/the number/quantity of sperm present

- ☐ Morphology: the size, shape, and structure of the sperm

- ☐ Motility: how well the sperm move

Semen Analysis

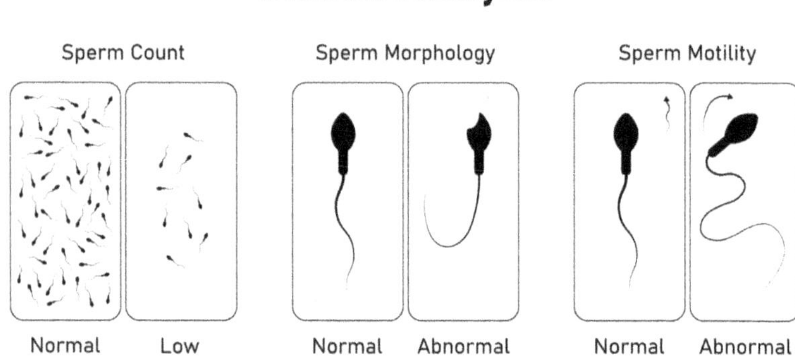

These factors are essential in determining the overall quality of the sperm, its potential to fertilise an egg and support healthy embryonic development.

When one of my patients receives a poor semen analysis result, the first thing I do is reassure them. It's important to understand that spermatogenesis (the process of sperm production) is dynamic and ongoing. With the right dietary, lifestyle, and supplement changes, significant improvements can be seen in just a few months in many cases.

But before treatment begins, we need to identify the root causes of poor sperm health. These vary widely. Some patients may be affected by one factor, others by several. Each case requires individual investigation and a tailored plan.

The bottom line is this: yes, your sperm can get better. I've seen it on countless occasions in my clinical practice. There are many effective tools available to support sperm health. So don't lose hope. Stick with me, and together we'll work through the steps that can lead to meaningful improvement.

Does age play a role in sperm quality?

Yes, age absolutely matters, but in a different way than it does for females.

For females, fertility tends to decline more sharply, often beginning in the mid-thirties. This is due to a limited number of eggs in the ovaries and the hormonal changes that come with age, especially around the perimenopausal transition. This is why egg freezing is often encouraged earlier in life.

Males, on the other hand, continue producing sperm throughout their lives. But that doesn't mean sperm quality stays the same forever. Starting in the late thirties, research shows a gradual decline in both sperm quality and quantity. Age has been identified as an independent factor that affects sperm health.

Here's the good news: you have far more control than you might think.

Unlike eggs, sperm are generated continuously. This means every few months, your body is producing a new batch, and you can influence the quality of that process. Nutrition, lifestyle habits, supplements, and targeted strategies all have a measurable impact. Everything outlined in this book is designed to help you take control of that process.

So, if you're in your forties or fifties and thinking about starting or growing your family, now is the time to act. Age may not be reversible, but the health of your sperm is something you can work on today. You have real power to improve your chances of conception and give your future child the best possible start.

Before jumping into IVF, let's make sure IVF works

If your semen analysis has come back with poor results, or you've been told that IVF or ICSI is your best option, this chapter is especially important for you. IVF and ICSI are incredible technologies that have given millions of couples the chance to become parents. Still, their success depends heavily on the quality of the sperm and the egg. That's why doing the preparation work beforehand is so valuable. Preconception care gives your body the time it needs to create a healthier batch of sperm and improve outcomes when IVF is your best option.

STRUCTURE OF A SPERM

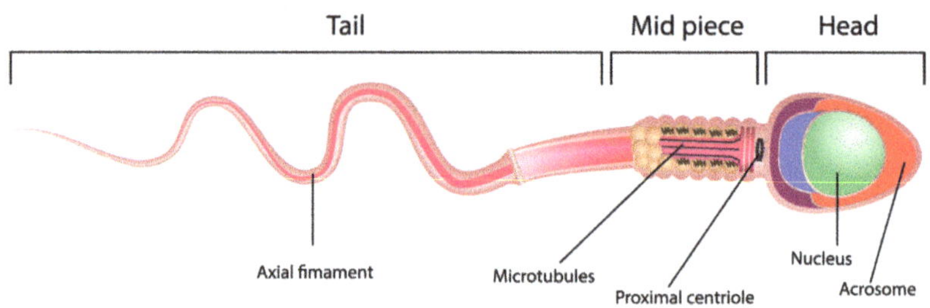

In many cases of male-factor infertility, ICSI is offered as the main solution. This technique allows an embryologist to select a sperm that appears to have the best shape and motility, then inject it directly into the egg.

But here's the limitation: no matter how skilled the embryologist, they cannot see what truly matters most, which is the DNA inside the nucleus of the sperm. The twenty-three chromosomes that carry the genetic instructions are invisible under the microscope.

This is where a DNA fragmentation panel becomes so important. Unlike a standard semen analysis, which looks only at the surface level factors like count, morphology and movement, this test examines the integrity of the DNA inside the nucleus of the sperm. If fragmentation is high, the sperm may fertilise the egg, but the embryo is unlikely to develop normally. It may stop growing in the lab, fail to implant in the uterus, or result in early miscarriage, usually within the first weeks of pregnancy. We'll explore DNA fragmentation in more detail in a later chapter, but it is a test that should always be considered when assessing sperm health.

Let me be clear: this is not about rejecting IVF or ICSI. Many of my patients would not have their children without these remarkable technologies. I am strongly in favour of using them when they are truly needed. What I am saying is that IVF should not be seen as a shortcut that makes sperm quality irrelevant. IVF will have a much higher success rate if the quality of the sperm has been maximised through optimal preconception care. If the DNA is damaged, no technology can repair it.

This is why preconception care is so powerful. Lifestyle, nutrition, exercise, and targeted supplementation can not only improve sperm count, motility, and morphology, but they can also reduce DNA fragmentation and protect the genetic material carried inside each sperm cell. That means healthier embryos, higher implantation rates, and fewer heartbreaking disappointments.

Think of the three months before IVF as a training camp. Spermatogenesis takes seventy-two to seventy-four days. By treating this period as if you and your partner are already pregnant, you give yourselves the best possible chance of success.

Doing this as a couple is especially motivating. Many females have already committed to these changes, but when their partners join the results can be profound. IVF and ICSI success rates can increase dramatically.

Current trends and statistics: let's be realistic

Sperm quality and quantity have been declining for decades. This isn't an exaggeration; it is a well-documented phenomenon. Understanding this trend gives us perspective and, more importantly, the power to act.

A comprehensive global review looked at 223 studies, including sperm samples from more than 57,000 males across 53 countries, collected between 1973 and 2018. The findings showed a clear trend:

- Average sperm concentration dropped by 51% from 1973 to 2018.

- Before the year 2000, the average annual decline was about 1.16%

- After 2000, the rate more than doubled to 2.64% per year.

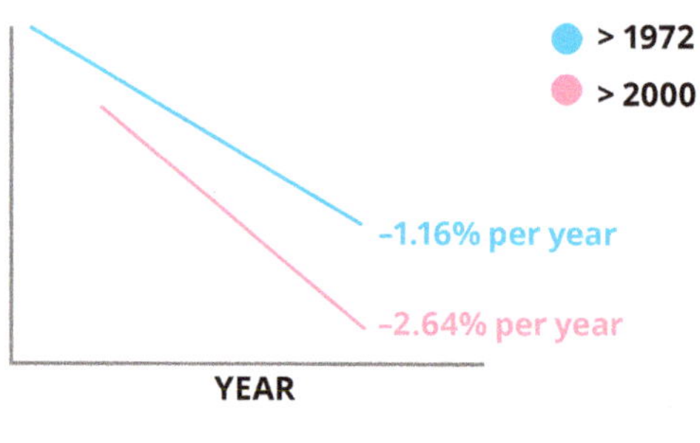

(Levine et al., 2023)

This shows us that while sperm health has been declining for decades, the pace of decline has accelerated in recent years. Researchers point to several contributing factors, such as exposure to environmental toxins, hormone-disrupting chemicals, sedentary lifestyles, obesity, smoking, and poor dietary patterns.

The researchers concluded:

> "This substantial and persistent decline is now recognized as a significant public health concern. In 2018, a group of leading clinicians and scientists called for governments to acknowledge decreased male fertility as a major public health problem and to recognize the importance of male reproductive health for the survival of the human (and other) species."

More information = More power

Now that we've looked at the current trends in sperm health and the crucial role of the male factor in fertility, it's time to focus on the bright side.

There is a lot you can do to change your fertility outcomes, and I'm here to guide you through it.

Together, we'll use the best available research, backed by years of clinical experience working with males and couples, to help you make real, effective changes.

You'll learn how to integrate practical strategies into your daily routine. Step by step, these changes will support your body in producing healthier, stronger sperm. In just a few months, your sperm quality and quantity can look completely different.

Chapter 3

Understand your hormones: beyond testosterone

Before we discuss treatments, supplements, or lab results, you'll need to understand how your reproductive system works. Knowledge gives you options, it allows you to take control of your fertility with confidence.

In my clinical practice, I focus on education, not just instructions. I explain what's happening and why. When patients understand their own bodies, they're more motivated, more consistent, and more successful.

Let's break down how sperm is made, how hormones drive the process, and why it matters for your fertility.

MALE REPRODUCTIVE HORMONES

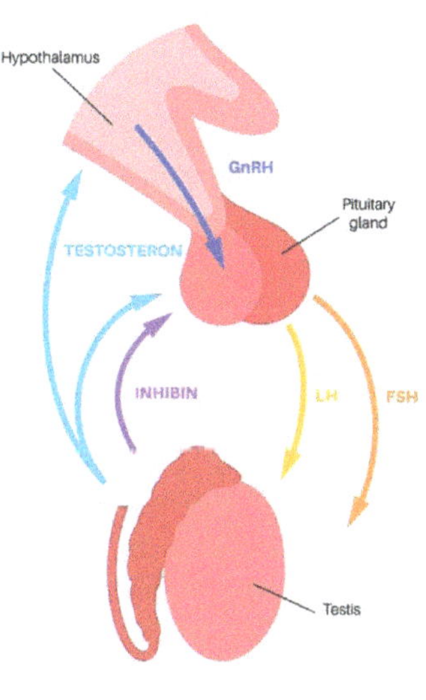

How your brain and testes communicate

Sperm production doesn't happen in isolation. It is controlled by a sophisticated communication system between your brain and your testes. When this system runs smoothly, hormone levels remain balanced, and sperm production is supported. But when it is disrupted, testosterone can decline, and fertility can be compromised.

The brain releases two key hormones that target the testes:

- ☐ FSH, or follicle stimulating hormone travels to the testes and activates the cells that start and maintain sperm production (Sertoli cells).

- ☐ LH, or luteinising hormone, also travels to the testes and stimulates specific cells to produce testosterone (Leydig cells).

The feedback loop: keeping hormones in balance

Communication between the brain and the testes works through a negative feedback loop. When testosterone or sperm production rises, signals are sent back to the brain to reduce stimulation; when levels fall, the brain increases LH or FSH release again.

As sperm production increases, the testes release inhibin, a hormone that signals the brain to reduce FSH. Likewise, when testosterone levels rise, the brain responds to the higher testosterone levels by lowering LH production. This continuous feedback keeps hormone levels stable and ensures sperm are produced at a healthy, steady rate, not too fast and not too slow.

Testosterone and sperm maturation

Testosterone plays a crucial role in sperm maturation. Inside the testes, testosterone acts directly on the Sertoli cells, guiding the transformation of developing sperm cells into fully mature and functional sperm. Without adequate testosterone, this process slows or becomes incomplete, leading to a higher proportion of immature sperm that are less capable of fertilising an egg. This is one of the most important, yet often overlooked, factors in male fertility.

When testosterone levels are low, sperm quality and maturity are noticeably reduced.

Raul Pastrana

Beyond sperm health, testosterone plays several vital roles throughout the body. It supports muscle strength, bone density, and energy levels, while also influencing motivation, confidence, and sex drive. When testosterone levels are optimal, male patients often report clearer thinking, better mood regulation, and a stronger sense of well-being.

Maintaining healthy testosterone levels is therefore essential for not only sperm maturation and fertility but also for overall physical and mental health.

When the system falls out of balance

This hormonal balance is delicate and can easily be disrupted by various factors, one of the most common being stress.

Short-term stress can be beneficial. For example, the temporary stress of exercise encourages the body to adapt, leading to improved strength and endurance. But when stress becomes chronic, it interferes with the hormonal communication between the brain and the testes.

A good example is overtraining, something I frequently observe in clinical practice. Pushing the body beyond its recovery capacity leads to persistently elevated cortisol levels. This, in turn, suppresses LH release from the brain, which lowers testosterone production and ultimately affects sperm quality.

Stress isn't only physical. Poor sleep, long work hours, emotional strain, exposure to environmental toxins, and heavy metals all add pressure to the system. Over time, these signals tell the brain that the environment is not ideal for reproduction, and the body responds by slowing or reducing sperm production.

Spermatogenesis: sperm synthesis

Spermatogenesis is the complete cycle of sperm creation. It takes about seventy-two to seventy-four days for a sperm cell to fully mature and be ready for ejaculation. This means that the sperm you produce today reflects your choices and environment over the last three months.

Understanding this cycle is powerful because it shows how much influence you have. Every stage of sperm development is shaped by the nutrients you consume, the quality of your sleep, your level of physical activity, and your exposure to toxins. By making positive changes now, you are directly impacting the health of the sperm you will release in the months ahead.

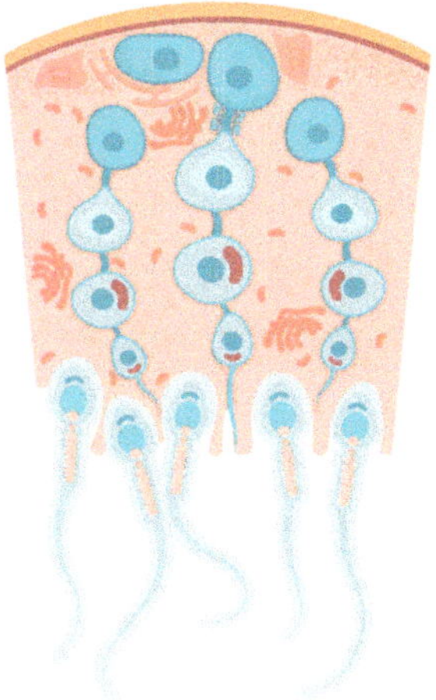

The good news is that sperm production responds well to positive changes. Here are the most important ways to support the process during the seventy-two-day cycle:

- ☐ Consistent, restorative sleep helps maintain balanced hormone signals.

- ☐ A nutrient-rich diet provides the building blocks for healthy sperm and protects them from cellular damage.

- ☐ Regular movement improves blood flow and hormone sensitivity while avoiding the setbacks that come with overtraining.

- ☐ Antioxidants, from both food and supplements, help safeguard sperm DNA as cells mature.

The last 15 days before ejaculation: why they matter the most

While the full sperm cycle in sperm synthesis is important, the last ten to fifteen days before ejaculation are especially critical. At this stage, the sperm are travelling through the epididymis. This is the long, coiled tube on top of and behind the testis, where sperm mature and gain motility. It is at this stage that sperm are highly susceptible to damage from oxidation and free radical damage.

Oxidative stress occurs when free radicals overwhelm your body's natural antioxidant defences, leading to damage in sperm DNA, morphology and motility. This lowers sperm quality and reduces the likelihood of a successful conception.

This applies to both natural conception and assisted reproduction or IVF. Whether you're trying to conceive at home, planning to freeze sperm, or preparing for treatments like IUI (intrauterine insemination) or ICSI, protecting your sperm during this window is essential.

This information becomes even more important if you are going to freeze sperm or provide a sample to fertilise the eggs collected during a stimulatory cycle for IVF or ICSI, as you have a real opportunity to maximise the quality of your sperm batch and obtain the best quality embryos. Following the core principles we've discussed, especially in the final fifteen days before collection. That short window can make a significant difference in the health and performance of the sperm you provide.

- ☐ Get consistent deep and restorative sleep.
- ☐ Avoid alcohol, smoking, and processed foods.
- ☐ Avoid overheating the testes (no saunas, tight clothing, sitting for long periods of time or cycling).
- ☐ Eat antioxidant-rich foods, such as berries, citrus, leafy greens, and nuts.
- ☐ Consider antioxidant supplementation.
- ☐ Ejaculation every two to three days

During this period, I often recommend high-dose vitamin C and NAC (n-acetyl cysteine). These supplements are well-researched and support the body's ability to protect sperm from damage.

<u>Testosterone is not the whole story</u>

Many male patients are told their testosterone levels are "normal" and therefore assume that means their sperm must also be healthy. This is one of the biggest misconceptions in male fertility. Testosterone and sperm are both produced in the testes, but by different types of cells. It's entirely possible to have healthy testosterone levels while still having a low sperm count, poor motility, or abnormal morphology.

This is why blood tests alone are not enough. Hormones provide valuable information, but they don't give the full picture. A semen analysis is essential to truly understand your fertility status.

That said, if your semen analysis comes back less than ideal, a follow-up blood test becomes even more important. It can reveal whether hormone imbalances are contributing to poor sperm health and provides another layer of insight into what could be happening within your reproductive system.

You now understand the basics of your reproductive system, the role of hormones, and how sperm are produced. Most importantly, you know that you have real influence over this process. In the next chapter, we'll look in detail at the tests that matter most, both semen and blood, and how to interpret them so you know exactly where you stand and what actions to take next.

You are already ahead of the curve. Keep going.

Getting an accurate assessment of your case will determine your chances of success and improvement. It is essential to identify the cause (or causes) leading to poor sperm health. Nothing will improve by taking a fancy supplement you found online with great reviews or using a product or strategy that worked well for your friend or someone else.

If you don't address YOUR cause for your poor sperm health, YOUR chances of conception will not increase.

Raul Pastrana

Semen analysis:
instructions, parameters, reference ranges and interpretation

Instructions

Before doing a semen analysis, it's essential to understand that certain variables can impact your results, sometimes significantly.

To ensure your results are as accurate and representative as possible, please follow these preparation guidelines carefully. The goal is to minimise any external influences that could skew the results.

Abstinence

Two to four days of complete abstinence are recommended before collecting the sample. I always advise my patients to aim for three days. This is something we can repeat in the future if a second analysis is required to understand the progress of treatment. By testing under the same conditions, we can truly compare apples with apples.

Shortened abstinence periods (less than two days) can lead to:

- o **Reduced volume and sperm count:** A shorter interval between ejaculations often means the testes haven't had enough time to produce and accumulate an optimal number of mature sperm, leading to a lower sperm count.

- o **Potential lower motility:** Too frequent ejaculation can impact motility. While research isn't entirely conclusive, I have found this to be true in my clinical practice.

Higher abstinence (more than four days) can lead to:

- o Increase volume and sperm count: Allowing more time between ejaculations can result in a high volume and total sperm count.

- o Decline in sperm quality: Although your quantity may be higher, sperm motility and morphology can decrease because older sperm are more susceptible to oxidative damage and reduced vitality over time.

Deliver your sample onsite

Yes, I understand how obtaining the sample in your home and getting it to the lab may seem like an easier and more comfortable option, but again, you are spending a few hundred dollars to get this test done, so it is important to ensure you receive accurate results.

For this, it is better to provide the sample onsite at the clinic or testing facility, as it ensures immediate processing under controlled conditions. This reduces the chance of temperature variations and delays, which can significantly affect motility, viability and overall quality.

If providing the sample onsite isn't possible, there are a few things I want you to consider when collecting and delivering the sample:

o   Body temperature: Keep the sample as close to body temperature as possible (thirty-seven degrees). This prevents sudden temperature changes that can damage the sperm cells. Simply keep the container inside your pocket, close to your skin.

o   Insulated Container: If you are travelling long distances, consider placing the sample in a small, insulated bag

o   Delivery within sixty minutes: aim to deliver the sample within one hour of collection to minimise quality loss. The sooner it is delivered, the better.

Ensure hydration

His may sound like an obvious one, but important to mention, nonetheless. Dehydration, even for a short period of time, will lead to a decrease in semen volume.

Delay the test if you have experience recent illness: As we have explained, the process of spermatogenesis is extremely sensitive. If your body has been fighting a bacterial or viral infection, if you have had food poisoning or any other recent illness, it can compromise the quality of the sperm. Therefore, it would be better to delay the collection of the sample:

o   For mild illness without fever, waiting seven to ten days after symptoms have fully resolved is sufficient.

- o For more severe illness with fever, it is generally better to wait for a complete spermatogenesis cycle (seventy-two to seventy-four days) before collecting the sample.

In practice, I give my patients a specific timeframe depending on their unique circumstances. Sometimes waiting three months for the collection isn't possible; in cases like this, I will provide them with antioxidants and compounds to protect the testes and the production of sperm.

Parameters and reference ranges

When you receive the results from your semen analysis, the main parameters assessed include:

Semen Volume: millilitres of semen produced during one ejaculation.

Sperm Concentration or Sperm Count: the number of sperm per 1 ml of sample.

Total Sperm Number: total number of sperm in the ejaculated sample.

Motility parameters:

- o *Progressive Motility:* the percentage of sperm moving forward. This is the type of sperm capable of reaching the egg in natural conception, as it needs to travel all the way to the fallopian tubes to meet the egg.

- o *Non- progressive motility:* percentage of sperm moving but not in a meaningful direction

- o *Immotile sperm:* sperm that do not move at all.

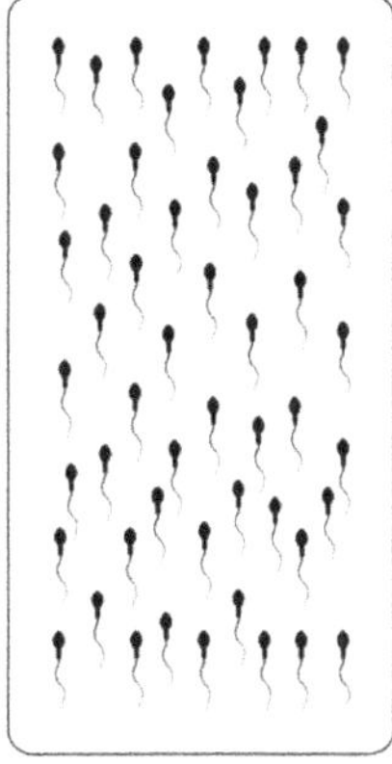
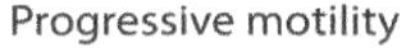

Progressive motility

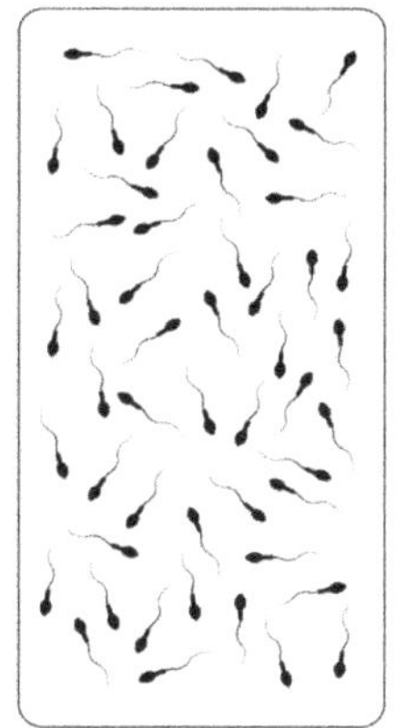

Non-progressive motility

<u>Morphology</u>: The percentage of sperm with normal shape, size and structure. This factor is of great importance if you are trying for natural conception. Poor morphology will negatively affect the capacity of the sperm to fertilise the egg.

Once you get your semen analysis results, comparing them to reference ranges is the key to understanding your fertility potential.

Interpretation understanding semen reference ranges

In 2010, the World Health Organisation (WHO) analysed semen data from more than 4,500 males across fourteen countries whose partners conceived within twelve months of trying. From this cohort, the WHO established the "reference ranges" that most laboratories still use today.

Here is what they did. Researchers ranked semen parameters such as sperm count, motility, and morphology. They then set the lower reference limit at the fifth percentile. In practical terms, this means that the bottom five percent of participants in the study were used to define what is considered "normal."

Think carefully about what that means. If your semen analysis falls close to the current reference range, you are being compared with those who had the lowest sperm quality in the study, but still managed to conceive. In fact, 95 percent of the males in that research had better results, and it's likely that most males with this low result are not able to achieve natural conception.

This is a little like comparing yourself to the students who just scraped through an exam. Passing with the lowest grade does not mean you are performing at your best. It simply means you met the minimum to get by. For fertility, aiming for the middle or even the top of the group makes far more sense if you want the best chances of success.

Distribution of semen examination results from men in couples starting a pregnancy within one year of unprotected sexual intercourse leading to a natural conception.

From Campbell et al. (5); fifth percentile given with variability (95% confidence interval)

Parameter (units)	N	Centile									
		2.5th	5th	(95% CI)	10th	25th	50th	75th	90th	95th	97.5th
Semen volume (ml)	3586	1.0	1.1	(1.3-1.5)	1.8	2.3	3.0	4.2	5.5	6.2	6.9
Sperm concentration (million/ml)	3587	11	16	(15-18)	22	36	66	110	166	208	254
Total sperm number (million per ejaculate)	3584	29	39	(35-40)	58	108	210	363	561	701	865
Progressive motility (PR, %)	3389	24	30	(29-31)	36	45	55	63	71	77	81
Non-progressive motility (NP, %)	3387	1	1	(1-1)	2	4	8	15	26	32	38
Immotile spermatozoa (IM, %)	2800	15	20	(19-20)	23	30	37	45	53	58	65
Vitality (%)	1337	45	51	(50-56)	60	69	78	88	95	97	98
Normal forms (%)	3335	3	4	(3.9-4.0)	5	8	11	23	32	39	45

Source: WHO laboratory manual for the examination and processing of human semen, Sixth Edition (2021).

The 50th percentile represents the median. Half of the participants in the study scored above it and half below. Reaching this level already gives you a stronger chance of conceiving.

If your results are near or below the fifth percentile, this does not mean conception is impossible, but it does mean it is probably going to be more difficult, take longer and less likely to occur. It strongly indicates there's significant room for improvement. The encouraging part is that sperm health is highly adaptable. As we've discussed, with the right combination of lifestyle changes, nutrition, supplementation, and targeted treatment, semen quality can improve in just a few months.

DNA fragmentation

Remember the structure of sperm. The head contains the nucleus with the 23 chromosomes. If fertilisation is adequate, it will combine with the 23 chromosomes from the egg to create the DNA unique for each baby.

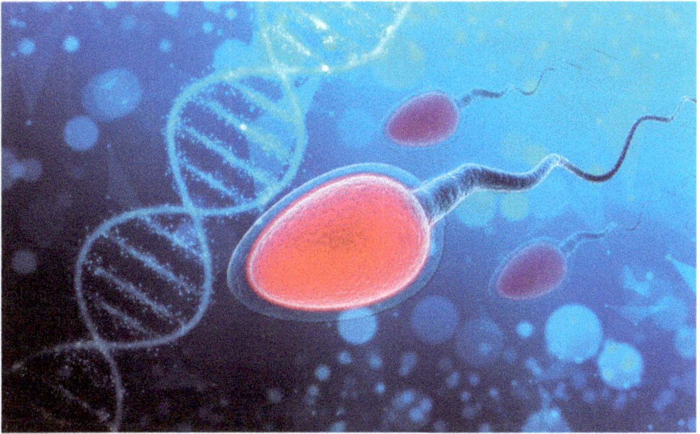

The chromosomes in the nucleus can become damaged due to multiple factors, such as:

- Increased oxidation and inflammation: smoking and alcohol

- Chronic infections: bacterial, viral or STIs

- Heat exposure: tight underwear, saunas, cycling or sitting for long periods of time.

- Lack in key nutrients required for DNA stability: omega-3, folate, zinc, selenium and CoQ10
- Environmental exposures: microplastics, pesticides and heavy metals
- Advanced paternal age
- Very frequent ejaculation or prolonged abstinence

Yes, many factors can damage the genetic material inside the head of the sperm.

A standard semen analysis doesn't give any information regarding the quality and the integrity of the genetic material. To obtain this information, you will need to get a **DNA fragmentation panel**. This test will allow you to know the average percentage of sperm in your sample that have damaged or fragmented DNA. The lower the DNA fragmentation result, the higher the quality and integrity of your sperm.

How to interpret your results based on the DNA Fragmentation Index (DFI)

DFI percentage	Interpretation	Impact on fertility
< 15%	Normal	Low risk of fertility issues. Good sperm DNA integrity.
15-25%	Moderate DNA fragmentation	Some risk of infertility, reduced embryo quality, and miscarriage. Some studies show significant reduction in IVF embryo quality and successful rates with DNA fragmentation above 20%.
> 25%	High DNA fragmentation	Higher risk of infertility, poor embryo development, failed IVF/ICSI, and miscarriage.
> 30-40%	Very high DNA fragmentation	Significant fertility challenges, increased risk of IVF/ICSI failure, and miscarriage.

Based on my clinical experience, to obtain the best fertility outcomes, it is better to aim for a DNA fragmentation under 10%, the lower the better, and often I will see my patient's results come back very low (<5%) after appropriate treatment and health improvement.

- What happens if your DNA fragmentation result is elevated?

There are many effective ways to reduce the percentage of fragmented DNA.

You can alter your diet to increase antioxidants and reduce toxins to decrease free radical damage. You can avoid alcohol, smoking, vaping, recreational drugs, and unnecessary pharmaceutical medication (under the supervision of your health care provider) during the three months before conception.

We will explore treatment options and other strategies in later chapters, but I can already tell you there are many tools you can implement in your daily life to improve this parameter.

If your first test result came back showing a high DNA fragmentation, don't be discouraged; this is just a baseline level. By applying the principles outlined in later chapters, you will be able to improve your numbers and increase the chances of conception, whether naturally or through IVF.

- DNA fragmentation and early miscarriage

It's a common misconception that if a couple can conceive but experiences an early miscarriage, the cause must lie with the female side. This assumption places too much responsibility on the female partner, when in many cases it isn't accurate. One important factor that is often overlooked is sperm DNA fragmentation.

Semen with high DNA fragmentation can still fertilise an egg. Implantation may even occur. But as the embryo starts to grow, it becomes increasingly dependent on the integrity of the DNA contributed by both the egg and the sperm.

Raul Pastrana

If the sperm has damaged DNA, this can lead to embryo chromosomal abnormalities that interfere with development. As a result, the embryo may stop growing. This typically happens between weeks six and ten of pregnancy, when the cells are dividing rapidly and beginning to form early structures. The body may then respond by naturally ending the pregnancy, resulting in a miscarriage or an early pregnancy loss.

This issue is particularly relevant in cases of ICSI. During ICSI, the sperm is selected based on how it looks and moves (morphology and motility), but these visual characteristics don't show the DNA quality. If a selected sperm carries fragmented DNA, the embryo may fail to reach the blastocyst stage, or it may implant and stop developing shortly after.

In short, high levels of sperm DNA fragmentation can result in infertility, increased time to conception, IVF and ICSI failure, poor embryo quality, miscarriage, birth defects, or even long-term health and cognitive issues in offspring.

DNA fragmentation and PGT testing.

Preimplantation genetic testing (PGT) is performed to screen embryos for genetic abnormalities in the 23 pairs of chromosomes before transfer. This testing can only be performed once the embryos have reached day 5 to 7 of embryo development (blastocyst).

Why is this important? In many cases, I have seen female patients use their frozen eggs with their partner's sperm for ICSI. Sometimes, this combination can result in several embryos failing PGT testing, meaning the egg and sperm chromosomes together create a DNA blueprint that cannot support a healthy, viable baby. It can also lead to embryos that fail to develop at all, have poor quality, or do not reach the blastocyst stage, the important developmental stage we aim to achieve by day 5 before the embryo is transferred into female partner.

Women go through a huge amount of effort to obtain those eggs. For men, obtaining sperm is a very quick, mechanical process that can be done within minutes. By following the preconception strategies outlined in later chapters, you can significantly improve the quality of your sperm, and in turn, give the remaining eggs your partner has (whether frozen or still in the ovaries) a stronger chance of creating life.

Preconception care always applies to both partners.

Raul Pastrana

Note: There are many types of PGT screening, such as PGT-A, PGT-M and PGT-SR. It is out of the scope of this book to understand the differences and relevance between these. However, the principles to improve outcomes on any of these tests remain equally important and relevant.

Chapter 5

Blood test: your hormones are important

To improve the quality of your semen, it is essential to understand which factors are affecting your spermatogenesis. This requires looking at a few key blood parameters and hormones that, in my practice, are non-negotiable and need to be investigated for every individual wishing to conceive. Improving these markers will lead to significant benefits for the well-being of the person making the changes (sleep, stress, longevity, gut health, etc), pregnancy outcomes and the health of your future baby.

Let's start with the hormones associated with the male reproductive system:

Hormone	Function	Reference Range	Optimal Reference Range
LH (Luteinizing hormone)	Stimulate specialised cells in the testes (Leydig Cells) to produce Testosterone	1.5 to 9.3 IU/L	3 to 6/8 IU/L
FSH (Follicle Stimulating Hormone)	Stimulate specialised cells in the testes (Sertoli Cells) to produce sperm.	1.5 to 12.4 IU/L	2 to 4/6 IU/L
Total Testosterone	Total amount of Testosterone produced by the testes	10 to 30 nmol/L	>15 - 30 nmol/L
Oestrogen	Important hormone for reproduction, mood, cognition and libido	40 to 115 pmol/L	50 to 120 pmol/L
Prolactin	Involved in testosterone and reproductive health	73 to 306 mIU/L	<150 mIU/L

These are some of the key hormones involved in male reproductive health. None of them work in isolation. Each one interacts with the others in a complex system. Understanding the basics empowers you to ask better questions and request the right tests from your health practitioner (doctor or naturopath).

When it comes to checking your hormones, timing really matters. Testosterone follows a daily rhythm, peaking in the morning and gradually declining throughout the day. That's why it is so important to test testosterone first thing in the morning. I've seen plenty of results that looked "low" simply because the sample was taken in the afternoon, when testosterone levels are naturally lower.

Another factor that can affect your results is recent illness. Even something as mild as a cold or flu can temporarily suppress testosterone. If you've been unwell, it's always better to wait at least two to three weeks after you've fully recovered before having your blood taken. This way, you'll get a more accurate picture of your real baseline when your body is working at its best.

If any of your results fall outside the ideal range, take that as a signal to look deeper, not as a reason to panic. A naturopath or functional medicine doctor who takes a comprehensive, whole-body approach can help you understand your unique situation. With the right care and guidance, you can achieve hormonal balance and improve your fertility outcomes.

Why you should test free testosterone

When testosterone is tested, it is vital to check both free testosterone and total testosterone. Total testosterone reflects how much of this hormone your testes are producing. However, not all of your testosterone can produce an effect in your body. A significant portion is "tied up" to a protein called SHBG (sex hormone binding globulin); this portion of testosterone cannot exert its effects in the body.

Only the free testosterone, the portion unattached to the SHBG protein, can bind to testosterone receptors throughout the body and create its effects. Free testosterone is responsible for sex drive, muscle strength, energy levels, mental focus and of course sperm production.

To gain a clear understanding of your hormonal health and testicular function, you need both assessments: free testosterone and total testosterone.

Free Testosterone = Total Testosterone – Testosterone bounded to SHBG

Your thyroid should also be tested

When we think about male fertility, testosterone is the hormone which steals the spotlight. But there's another key player that's often overlooked: thyroid hormones.

The thyroid is a small gland in your neck that acts like a control centre for your metabolism. It helps regulate mood, energy, weight and your reproductive and testicular function.

Even though thyroid problems are more common amongst females, males can also experience imbalances. And when the thyroid isn't working properly, it can quietly affect sperm quality, testosterone levels, libido and even mental health.

These are the most important parameters regarding thyroid function:

Test name	Function	Reference Range	Optimal Reference Range
TSH (Thyroid Stimulating Hormone)	This hormone is created in your brain and travels to your thyroid to stimulate the production of Thyroid Hormones T3 & T4	0.5 to 4.5 mIU/L	1 to 2.5 mIU/L
T4	The main hormone produced by the thyroid gland	10 to 20 pmol/L	
T3	The active form of thyroid hormone, concerted from T4	3.1 to 6.8 pmol/L	
TPO Antibodies	Autoimmune marker	< 35 to 60 IU/mL	< 35 IU/mL
TG Antibodies	Autoimmune marker	< 20 IU/mL	

If, after testing any of these hormones, your levels are out of the reference ranges, it's vital to follow up with a health care provider. They can help you understand what the best course of action is to improve your thyroid function.

Homocysteine, B12 and folate

Homocysteine is one of my favourite blood markers. It provides insight into inflammation levels, nutrient status, and overall metabolic health, all of which are directly linked to sperm quality and reproductive outcomes.

Homocysteine is an amino acid that builds up in the blood when the body lacks certain nutrients, particularly activated folate (5-MTHF) and vitamin B12. When levels are too high, homocysteine becomes inflammatory and can affect blood vessels, circulation, and cellular function.

Elevated homocysteine levels or hyperhomocysteinemia has been associated with:

- reduced sperm concentration and motility.
- increased DNA fragmentation.
- erectile dysfunction.
- compromised blood flow to the testes.
- higher oxidative stress, which impairs sperm development.

Even if a semen analysis looks normal, elevated homocysteine can quietly reduce the chances of successful conception. It can even affect embryo quality by increasing DNA fragmentation.

In Australia, the general reference range for homocysteine is five to fifteen micromoles per litre (µmol/L). This range reflects population-wide averages, rather than fertility-specific goals.

For males trying to optimise fertility, I prefer to see homocysteine levels between six and eight µmol/L. This narrower range supports better/ healthier/improved DNA methylation, hormone function, and sperm production.

Common reasons for elevated homocysteine include:

- deficiency in folate, vitamin B12, or vitamin B6.
- specific genes: MTHFR.
- smoking.
- high alcohol intake.
- chronic inflammation.
- liver stress or sluggish detoxification pathways.

The good news is that homocysteine is easy to improve/is one of the easiest markers to improve. In most cases, nutritional support with active forms of B vitamins such as methylated folate, methylcobalamin (B12), and pyridoxal-5-phosphate (B6) can reduce homocysteine to optimal levels. Addressing lifestyle habits like diet, alcohol intake, and smoking is also highly effective.

B12 and folate

	Reference Range	Optimal reference range for fertility
Folate	7 to 40 nmol/L	> 40 nmol/L
B12	80 to 340 nmol/L	>500 nmol/L
Active B12	38 to 75 nmol/L	>100 nmol/L

Iron

Iron is an essential nutrient in our diets. It is responsible for transporting oxygen in the red blood cells throughout our body. However, as with many cases, too much of a good thing can become harmful. Iron is also a heavy metal, and excess levels can lead to inflammation and oxidation. The liver and the testes are particularly vulnerable to the damage caused by high levels of oxidative stress associated with high levels of iron.

Poor sperm health has been associated with high levels of iron.

Raul Pastrana

Ferritin is the blood marker used to determine your iron reserves. If ferritin is sitting above 200 - 300 ug/L, it is a clear indication that this could be a barrier affecting sperm health. Interpreting iron studies is complex, and you should always review with an experienced functional medicine practitioner to fully understand what the patterns in your iron studies indicate.

Zinc

Zinc is a very important nutrient for reproduction and sperm health. Zinc is required for cell division during the process of spermatogenesis, being a key mineral for the structural integrity of sperm. This mineral is also required for testosterone synthesis.

Low levels of zinc have been associated with poor sperm health (poor motility and quantity).

Raul Pastrana

To determine whether you need to increase zinc consumption in your diet or supplementation, it is always best to do a blood test for Plasma Zinc. The Australian Reference ranges for plasma zinc are 9 to 19 umol/L. I prefer to see my patients sit between 13 to 18umol/L for sperm and testosterone optimisation.

Vitamin D

Vitamin D plays an important role in male reproductive health. Beyond supporting bone strength, immunity, and hormone balance, research indicates that it also affects how the testes function and sperm development. Both the testes and sperm cells contain vitamin D receptors and enzymes that activate the vitamin, suggesting vitamin D helps to regulate testosterone production and spermatogenesis.

Studies have shown that when vitamin D levels fall outside the normal range, sperm quality can be negatively affected. Both low (< 50 nmol/L) and high (> 125 nmol/L) levels of Vitamin D have been linked to poorer sperm concentration, motility, and morphology, as well as disruptions in hormonal balance.

Progressive motility, the sperm's ability to move forward effectively, appears to be the parameter most consistently impacted. However, other factors such as concentration and morphology may also be influenced.

Parameter	Vitamin D < 50 nmol/L	Vitamin D 50–125 nmol/L	Vitamin D > 125 nmol/L (n = 20)
Sperm concentration (million/mL)	52.1	84.0	46.7
Progressive motility (%)	45.5	52.6	38.4
Normal sperm heads (%)	20.1	27.4	18.0
Total progressive motile sperm count (million)	45.3	98.8	52.3
Total sperm count (million)	85.1	178.6	110.2

(Adapted from Hammoud et al., 2012)

Maintaining vitamin D levels within the middle range supports optimal outcomes for sperm health. From a clinical perspective, I generally aim for my patients' vitamin D levels to sit around 100 nmol/L, as this range is associated with the most balanced hormonal and sperm parameters.

The only reliable way to achieve this is by starting with a blood test to determine your baseline. If levels are low, supplementation and responsible sun exposure where possible can then be tailored to gradually reach a level closer to 100 nmol/L. Beginning supplementation without knowing your starting point can be counterproductive, as both high and low levels of vitamin D levels can be harmful for sperm health, as shown in the table, where extremes on either end correlated with poorer sperm parameters.

I use different forms of vitamin D, depending on an individuals levels and history of deficiency or responsiveness to supplementation, as some of us have a genetic predisposition to poor absorption.

There are many other blood and functional tests I employ to best understand the many varied ways in which your health and genetic predisposition are affecting your fertility. Ultimately, the more we know about your circumstances, the easier it is to achieve the results you're after. Nothing wastes time when trying to conceive more than not addressing the underlying factors delaying your time to conception.

Book a consultation using the link below if you would like personalised guidance on which tests are most appropriate for you, or support interpreting your results so you can implement the right treatment strategy and lifestyle changes to optimise your outcomes.

Make your booking here

Navigating the conventional medical model of fertility: fertility clinics, urologists and endocrinologists

When fertility becomes a challenge, many couples naturally turn to the medical system for support. This may include working with general practitioners, endocrinologists, urologists, and fertility specialists - each bringing valuable expertise to the process. However, it's important to approach this journey with awareness and to understand how best to navigate the system for your individual needs.

The fertility field has expanded rapidly in recent years, offering great advances in technology and access to treatment. Yet, alongside this growth, some patients describe feeling as though their care progressed very quickly, sometimes before they had the opportunity to explore underlying factors or prepare their bodies for conception. This doesn't mean the care they received was wrong; rather, it underscores how unique each fertility journey can be.

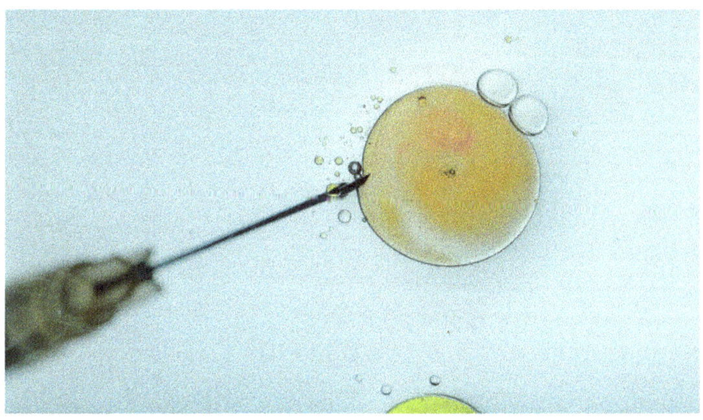

In my clinical experience, preparation often matters as much as the procedure itself. Preconception care still plays a crucial role, even when assisted reproductive techniques (ART) such as IVF are involved. These procedures can have significant physical, emotional, hormonal, and financial demands. That's why I often compare fertility preparation to training for a marathon; you wouldn't suddenly attempt to run over forty kilometres without training. Instead, you'd spend time preparing your body, nourishing it well, and gradually building resilience so that you have the best chance of success.

Allowing time to strengthen sperm and egg health beforehand can make a meaningful/considerable difference. A few months of focused preparation can help to reduce the side effects, support hormone balance, improve embryo quality, and sometimes even lead to natural conception before treatment begins; a scenario I have seen many times in practice. While there are never guarantees, couples who invest in preconception health often experience smoother cycles and better outcomes.

For males, this process begins with proper testing, a comprehensive semen analysis, including DNA fragmentation, alongside a detailed blood panel to assess hormones, nutrient levels, and inflammation. With that information, targeted changes can be made to improve sperm health within a relatively short time frame.

Of course, not every situation allows for this level of preparation. In some cases, IVF must begin right away, and that is entirely valid. However, when time permits, supporting egg and sperm quality through nutrition, supplementation, rest, and lifestyle choices can be a valuable investment in the overall process and its outcomes.

Some clinics prioritise efficiency, which can be appropriate for many patients. However, for others, a slightly slower, more individualised approach can make all the difference. The key is to ask questions, seek clarity, and feel confident in the plan you and your healthcare team develop together, which often means focusing on health as well as medicine, and employing the support of professionals with experience in preconception healthcare, as well as those with required medical expertise.

This is not about questioning your doctor; it's about building a collaborative relationship grounded in communication and mutual understanding. You deserve to be informed, supported, and treated as an individual. When both partners are given the time and space to prepare well, the journey toward conception often feels more aligned, more manageable, and more hopeful.

Chapter 7

The 4 pillars of sperm health

Lifestyle influences: nutrition, exercise, sleep and stress

The foundations of good health: nutrition, movement, sleep, and stress management, aren't just about feeling good or living longer; they're also the core pillars of sperm health. Sperm may be microscopic, but they're incredibly sensitive, reflecting your overall metabolic, hormonal, and inflammatory balance. When you eat well, train smart, rest deeply, and manage stress effectively, you support optimal testosterone levels, sperm count, motility, morphology, and DNA integrity. But when these areas are neglected, oxidative stress, insulin fluctuations, inflammation and hormonal imbalances can create the perfect storm for poor sperm quality.

The healthier you are, the healthier your sperm.

Raul Pastrana

Nutrition

What you eat, when you eat, and how much you eat all play a powerful role in your fertility. But it is not only about the food itself. It is also about how you relate to food and the choices you make every day. Shifting that relationship is one of the most important steps you can take to improve your reproductive health.

In my clinical work, I have seen firsthand how different bodies respond to different diets. Some patients feel their best on a mostly plant-based approach, while others thrive when red meat is part of their intake. There is no single diet that works for everyone, which is why I do not believe in a one-size-fits-all approach.

That said, I can give you some clear principles to follow. They are the same foundations I share with my patients, and when applied consistently, they lead to better sperm quality, healthier hormones, and stronger overall well-being.

Caloric intake

I am not someone who usually promotes strict calorie counting, nor is it something I ask my patients to do long-term. However, in the short term, it can be an eye-opening educational tool. Tracking your food intake for just a few days can reveal how many calories you are actually consuming, as well as the balance of protein, fat, and carbohydrates in your diet.

Many free apps and websites make this process simple. I usually suggest calorie tracking only when I suspect someone is consistently under-eating or, on the other hand, consuming more than their body needs. Having this information allows us to make the right adjustments - small changes that can have a significant impact on hormone balance and sperm health.

You can easily estimate your ideal daily calorie intake using an online calculator such as www.calculator.net/calorie-calculator.html. All you need to enter is your current weight, height, age, and level of physical activity. The calculator will then give you an approximate number of calories to maintain your weight, gain muscle, or lose body fat.

> For example, if you are 37, weight 75Kg with 180cm tall and have a moderate level of physical activity.
>
> You will need around 2483 calories per day
> to maintain your weight

Why am I spending so much time on this?

Overeating or undereating can place significant stress for the body, which can affect your hormonal levels and sperm health significantly. Counting your calories isn't a must. But if you have never done it and are concerned about not meeting your dietary requirements, it may be beneficial.

Tracking your food for three to four days can provide a clear picture/snapshot of your average intake of protein, fat, and carbohydrates.

Let's now take a closer look at each macronutrient and how much of each you should aim for:

Protein

Protein in each meal is crucial for long-term health. Aim to provide the body with at least 30 grams of protein in each of your main meals. This supports balanced blood glucose levels, reduces hunger and provides all the amino acids required for spermatogenesis. Amino acids are the building blocks of protein and play key roles in cellular function, energy production and antioxidant defence; in other words, they keep us alive.

If you consume thirty grams of protein across three meals per day, you will reach a total of ninety grams of protein daily. This may be enough for some men, but not for most.

There are two more factors we need to consider when determining your protein requirements. Your current weight and your daily level of physical activity.

The higher your daily physical activity, the more protein you will need. For example, if someone spends eight hours a day in front of a desk, they will have lower calorie and protein requirements than someone who is physically active for the same duration.

Another important consideration is your weekly exercise routine. With those two factors in mind: your current weight and your overall energy expenditure, you can calculate your daily protein requirements

- 1.2 g per kg of body weight for **sedentary individuals** (little to no exercise)

- 1.4 g per kg of body weight for **moderate activity** (light workouts, no more than two work outs per week)

- 1.6–1.8 g per kg of body weight for **highly active individuals** (frequent strength training or physically demanding jobs)

- 2 g per kg of body weight **for athletes** with demanding jobs.

For example, if you are 37, weigh 75Kg, are 180cm tall and have a moderate level of physical activity:

75 x 1.4 = 105grams

You will need around 105 grams of protein per day.

The source of your protein is just as important as the amount you consume. From both research and clinical practice, I show that males experience better fertility and hormonal outcomes when their protein comes from a *variety* of sources rather than relying on just one type.

Combining animal and plant-based proteins ensures a broader and more complete profile of amino acids, which are essential for sperm production, hormone synthesis, and overall metabolic health. Reliable nutrient-dense options include eggs, lean meats, poultry, fish, legumes, nuts, seeds, collagen, and high-quality protein powders.

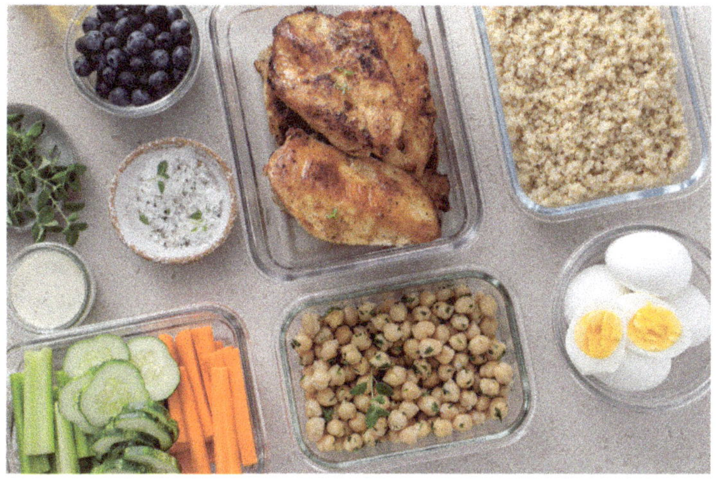

When it comes to fish, quality makes a difference. Wild-caught fish such as salmon, sardines, and anchovies are excellent sources of protein and omega-3 fatty acids, which play a key role in the structure of sperm cell membranes and reduce inflammation. Farmed fish, however, may carry higher levels of contaminants such as heavy metals (mercury) and persistent organic pollutants (including PCBs, microplastics and dioxins). Several studies have linked these compounds to reduced sperm quality and hormone disruption. In my practice, I have seen improvements in sperm health when patients reduce their intake of low-quality farmed fish and prioritise clean, nutrient-rich sources.

Fat

Fat is highly important for sperm health. Remember the structure of the sperm.

STRUCTURE OF A SPERM

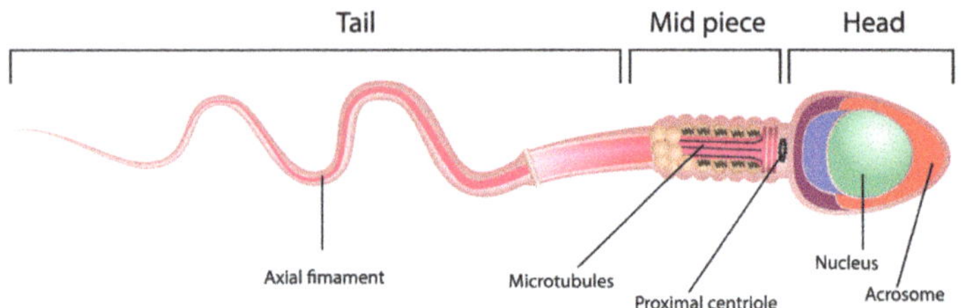

The head of the sperm contains the genetic material, made up of twenty-three chromosomes, which combine with the egg to form a healthy embryo. This head is surrounded by a lipid-rich membrane that is critical in protecting the DNA and supports the sperm's ability to fertilise the egg. A key component of this membrane is omega-3 fatty acids, which provide stability and flexibility to the cell structure.

Fats also play a crucial role in male fertility through hormone production. Cholesterol is the raw material used to synthesise testosterone in the testes. Without adequate fat intake, the body cannot produce sufficient testosterone, which is vital for normal sperm development, libido, and overall reproductive health.

Below are some of the principles I use with my patients when discussing fat consumption:

- Eat wild-caught fatty fish (salmon, sardines and anchovies)
- Include grass-fed meats and eggs
- Include avocado, nuts and seeds in moderation.
- Avoid trans fats and refined vegetable oils as they compete for omega-3 for absorption in the gut.
- Use olive oil, stored in a non-transparent container (dark glass or amber) and avoid plastic bottles. This ensures the oil retains all of its beneficial properties and nutrients while preventing oxidation from the light or the plastic.
- Coconut oil is also a good option in moderation while avoiding excess saturated fat intake, especially from grain-fed animal protein and deep-fried foods.

Omega-3 supplementation

In my clinical practice, I frequently recommend high-quality omega-3 supplements for patients aiming to boost sperm health. While a nutritious diet is essential, it can be challenging to obtain enough omega-3s from food alone, especially if you are trying to create noticeable improvements in a short time frame. Given that sperm production takes roughly seventy-two days, the window for improvement is limited, and supplementation can offer the extra support needed to optimise results.

Raul Pastrana

Fat should represent around 25 to 35% of your caloric intake.

For example, if you are 37, weight 75Kg are 180am tall and have a moderate level of physical activity.

Your total caloric intake to maintain weight should be around 2.483 calories per day

2.483 X 0.3 = 745 calories

There are 9 calories in each gram of fat.

745/9 = 83 g of fat per day

Carbohydrates

Carbohydrates have gained a bad reputation over the years. Many people think that eating carbs automatically leads to weight gain and poor health, so they try to avoid them altogether. In reality, carbohydrates are the body's main energy source. Inside the mitochondria, carbohydrates are converted into ATP (adenosine triphosphate), which powers nearly every function of the body, including muscle performance, brain activity, and sperm production.

The real issue is not carbohydrates themselves, but how much you eat and in what form. Modern Western diets tend to be high in refined carbohydrates and low in protein, which creating the perfect environment for fat gain, unstable blood sugar, and poor hormone balance.

Two key factors determine how many carbohydrates you should consume each day.

- Your activity level.

Physically active individuals and those who exercise regularly use more glucose for fuel. In contrast, individuals who live a more sedentary lifestyle generally require fewer carbohydrates.

- Your carbohydrate tolerance.

This varies widely between individuals and is strongly influenced by genetics. Some people can eat a high-carb diet without gaining weight or losing blood sugar control, while others are more sensitive and may see blood sugar spikes, cravings, fatigue, or weight gain with the same intake. This explains why one person may thrive on a higher-carb diet while another feels and performs better with fewer carbs.

Understanding both your activity level and your personal carbohydrate tolerance is key. Choosing whole-food carb sources such as vegetables, fruits, whole grains, and legumes, while limiting refined sugars and processed foods, will support better energy balance, hormone function, and overall sperm health.

The third consideration for carbohydrate intake is your desired outcome. When determining the percentage of calories you should obtain from carbohydrates based on your desired goal (such as weight loss, muscle gain, or maintenance), it's important to tailor it to your specific needs.

Here is a general guideline.

1. If you have high cholesterol, are carrying excess weight and need to reduce fat, carbohydrates need to be 30 to 40 % of your total calorie intake.

2. If you are healthy and are aiming to maintain your weight, carbohydrates should represent 45 to 55 % of your total calories.

3. If your goal is to gain muscle, you should consider increasing carbohydrate intake to 50 to 60 % of your total calories.

Most of your calories should come from complex carbohydrate sources rather than highly refined carbs. Good choices include sweet potato, potato, pumpkin, quinoa, rice, brown rice, buckwheat, legumes, and some healthy breads and pastas. Pre-cooking and cooling certain starchy foods, like potatoes, rice, or pasta, increases their resistant starch content. Resistant starch is not fully digested in the small intestine and instead reaches the colon, where it feeds beneficial gut bacteria. This promotes a healthy microbiome, improves gut health, and also helps with weight management by enhancing satiety and stabilising blood sugar.

Is organic really that important?

One of the questions I often hear from patients is: "Do I really need to eat everything organic?" My honest answer is no. Eating 100% organic is not realistic for most people. It can be expensive, time-consuming, and sometimes not even possible depending on where you live. But what I do recommend is choosing organic strategically.

Why does this matter for male fertility? Many conventionally grown foods contain pesticide residues, herbicides, and other environmental pollutants that can affect hormonal balance, reproductive health, and testicular function. These compounds can interfere with hormone production, damage sperm DNA, and reduce overall sperm quality. For example, studies have linked higher exposure to pesticides like organophosphates and glyphosates with lower testosterone levels and reduced sperm motility. Even low-level, repeated exposure can accumulate over time and place a significant burden on the body.

In my clinical experience, I have seen how making simple shifts toward cleaner food choices can improve outcomes. When we become more intentional about where our food comes from and invest in higher-quality produce, fertility parameters often improve within just a few months. These changes don't need to feel overwhelming.

It does not have to be all or nothing. Instead of aiming for perfection, the real goal is to make smarter choices where you can. Buying seasonal produce is often better both nutritionally and financially, since foods grown in season contain higher nutrient levels and usually cost less. For example, in Australia, this might mean enjoying mangoes, watermelon, and cucumbers in summer; apples, pears, and sweet potatoes in autumn; citrus fruits like oranges, mandarins, and grapefruits in winter; and vegetables such as asparagus, zucchini, and leafy greens in spring. Choosing what is naturally in season means fresher food, richer flavour, and better value for money.

Shopping at farmers' markets is another excellent option. Even if the produce isn't officially labelled organic, many small farmers use minimal chemicals and maintain better growing practices than large-scale suppliers. I also encourage my patients to explore vegetable box subscriptions or direct-from-farm delivery services. These options often cut out the supermarket middleman, meaning you receive fresher, higher-quality produce while supporting local growers. Not only does this improve the quality of your food, but it also supports small businesses in your community.

Think of these changes as another tool in your fertility toolkit. By lowering your exposure to harmful chemicals and prioritising fresher, more nutrient-dense foods, you are reducing unnecessary stress on the body and creating an environment where your hormones and sperm can thrive. The added benefit is that these habits support your long-term health well beyond fertility.

A final note

I really enjoy berries, especially blueberries. They are packed with antioxidants, taste great, and can be a fantastic addition to a diet focused on fertility. But as much as I like them, I always remind my patients that small, soft-skinned fruits like berries and grapes are more likely to carry higher levels of pesticides. Because their skin is so delicate, it is harder to wash chemicals off, which means choosing organic versions makes a real difference for fertility and overall health.

When it comes to cherries, I want to be completely open with you. Based on what I know about farming practices and how pesticides are commonly used on cherry crops, I personally choose not to eat them unless they are organic. This isn't something I can back with large clinical trials, but it is an informed belief I hold, and a guideline I feel comfortable sharing with my patients.

Raul Pastrana

Exercise

I've spent years working as a personal trainer, and I've seen exercise transform lives in ways that go far beyond the gym. It is not only about building muscle or losing weight. I've seen people sleep better, improve their energy, perform more confidently at work, and strengthen their relationships simply by moving their bodies more. These experiences shaped the way I practice today, because I know firsthand that exercise is one of the most powerful tools, we have for improving health and fertility.

For most of us, work is not optional. Sitting for eight hours a day is simply the reality of modern life, but that does not mean we have to accept the negative effects it has on hormones, cardiovascular health, and particularly sperm quality. The key is to find ways to move your body *around* your job.

This is not about becoming a super athlete or pushing yourself from zero to one hundred overnight. What matters are the small, sustainable changes that fit into daily life. Many of you reading this book may already be applying some of these strategies without even realising how beneficial they are for your fertility. Knowing that the habits you already practice, whether it is walking more, cycling to work, or lifting weights, are scientifically proven to support sperm health and testosterone can be incredibly motivating.

In this chapter, I will show you how these everyday changes, supported by science, can make a measurable difference to your health, your energy, and your fertility.

Walking

Engaging in regular walking routines, such as aiming for 10,000 steps per day, has been associated with several health benefits in males, including improved testosterone levels, enhanced sperm quality, better weight management and reduced risk of cardiovascular disease.

A 2021 study analysed the relationship between daily step count and serum testosterone levels in males. The results were conclusive: men with higher daily step counts had significantly higher testosterone levels and lower odds of hypogonadism (testosterone deficiency). The opposite was also true; those with the lowest step counts had a greater likelihood of poor testicular function.

If you are not sure how much you walk each day, start by checking your phone's health app or using a simple step counter. Once you know your baseline, the goal is not to jump straight to 10,000 steps a day. Instead, build up gradually. A helpful approach is to increase your daily step count by around 1,000 steps each week.

For example, if your average right now is 4,000 steps a day, aim for 5,000 the following week, then 6,000 the following week. Over time, you will build up to at least 10,000 steps a day, which is a solid foundation for supporting your cardiovascular health, hormone balance, and sperm function. This gradual increase is easier to stick with, less stressful on the body, and far more sustainable in the long run.

How you increase your step count will vary from person to person. For some, it may mean walking your dog more often or taking a 30-minute walk after lunch instead of staying at your desk. For others, it could be getting off public transport a stop earlier, parking further away from the office, or choosing stairs instead of the lift. Even small habits like pacing while on the phone or taking a short walk to clear your head before dinner can make a difference. The key is to find movement that fits naturally into your day, so it feels like part of your routine rather than an added chore.

Resistance training

Resistance training, simply put, is exercise where your muscles work against a form of resistance. This can be free weights, machines, resistance bands, or even your own bodyweight. In practical terms, it means going to the gym and doing strength-focused exercises.

Resistance training and regular movement are essential for long-term health. Preserving muscle mass and maintaining a healthy body composition are key factors for hormonal balance, sexual health, and male fertility. Muscle is not just about strength or appearance. It is one of the strongest predictors of how we age well. The ability to prevent muscle loss over time is the single most important factor in determining whether someone remains independent as they grow older. And the only way to preserve muscle is by stimulating it consistently through some form of resistance training.

Think about it this way: when someone is years old, their ability to stand up from a chair, walk comfortably, or continue to live independently will largely depend on whether they have maintained their muscle strength over the decades. I know this is slightly off topic, but it is worth mentioning because fertility is only one part of the bigger picture of lifelong health.

If you want to see a real transformation in your health, your fertility, and your overall quality of life, trust me when I say this: go to the gym three times a week for the next three months. You will be doing your part. Not only will your body start producing healthier sperm, but you will also be protecting your posture, strengthening your lower back, and preparing yourself for the years ahead. When you eventually become a parent and your child grows into a teenager, you will be older, but you will be fit enough to play sports, run, and share those experiences with them. Statistically, the healthier you are, the healthier your child is likely to be. You give them the best possible start through healthy sperm, but also by modelling that exercise is normal, valuable, and part of everyday life. They will learn this from you.

Okay, that got a bit emotional, so let's bring it back to science. Research shows that males who exercise for around seven hours per week have significantly better sperm parameters than those who exercise less than one hour per week. Seven hours is the upper end, but you don't need to reach that level to experience the benefits. As mentioned earlier, even three 45-minute sessions per week can create substantial improvements in testosterone levels, sperm production, and overall vitality.

On a physiological level, exercise improves cardiovascular health and blood flow throughout the body. Better circulation means more oxygen-rich blood and nutrients delivered to the testes, while waste products and oxidative stress are cleared more efficiently. This creates the ideal environment for sperm production.

The same improved circulation also supports erectile quality and frequency. Erections depend on healthy blood flow to the penis, and stronger circulation generally means stronger, longer-lasting erections. That translates directly into better sex, more confidence in the bedroom, and greater enjoyment in your relationship.

Cardio, running and cycling

Some of you reading this book may gravitate toward cardio as a main form of exercise, while others (myself included) prefer weights. The thing is, when it comes to long-term health and fertility, resistance training is generally more impactful than cardiovascular training; however, a well-balanced routine strategy should ideally include both. Saying that, I should also mention we are not aiming for perfection. My goal is to bring you well-rounded information about different types of exercises, their benefits and their potential downsides for fertility outcomes, so that you can make informed decisions.

I don't want you to feel that you need to suddenly start going to the gym, running, walking 10,000 steps a day, and attending yoga classes all at once to improve your fertility or sperm health. That's not the intention here. The message is simply that there are many different ways you can support your body and "do your part." As you read this section, I invite you to notice which strategies feel most realistic and achievable for your body, your needs, and your goals.

Running is a great way to increase your step count, raise your heart rate, and promote better blood flow throughout the body, including the testicular area. Health and fertility benefits linked to running can be seen after just a few months of moderate, steady routines like jogging. You don't need to run 10 km to experience results. Even short runs, around 3 km twice a week, can improve sperm quality, reduce DNA damage, and support healthier morphology.

That said, running is just one example of how raising your heart rate with cardiovascular exercise can benefit your health and fertility. If running isn't for you, there are many alternatives: brisk walking, swimming, rowing, cycling with the right adjustments, or even using an elliptical machine. The best form of cardio is the one you enjoy and can fit consistently into your lifestyle. Choose what works for you.

A note about cycling

I think cycling is a great way to stay active. However, when it comes to fertility, especially in the three months leading up to conception, it may be wise to limit long-distance rides. Extended time on the bike, combined with tight cycling wear, can increase scrotal temperature and create friction in the testicular area, both of which can affect sperm quality. If cycling is something you love, shorter sessions are generally fine, but for this critical preconception window, it's worth being extra cautious.

Raul Pastrana

Yoga and pilates

Yoga and Pilates are often overlooked by men, but they can be highly effective for both overall health and fertility. These practices build strength, improve flexibility, support posture, and increase body awareness. They may not look as intense as lifting heavy weights or running long distances, but they still provide resistance, improve circulation, and help regulate hormones, all of which are important factors in sperm health.

Reformer Pilates is particularly useful if you are dealing with joint concerns such as knee pain or arthritis. Because it is low-impact, it allows you to strengthen and challenge your muscles without putting unnecessary strain on your joints. This is one of the reasons why Pilates has become increasingly popular; it offers a genuine alternative to the traditional gym while still delivering real strength and mobility benefits.

Another reason I often recommend Yoga or Pilates is their impact on stress. As we've already discussed, chronic stress and elevated cortisol levels can interfere with testosterone production and sperm quality. If lab results and clinical signs, like insomnia, suggest that stress is a major factor affecting your health, these practices can be powerful tools. They require focused attention on posture and breathing, which naturally shifts your mind away from racing thoughts and into the present moment. For many men, this break in the stress cycle is exactly what their body needs. Adding just two to three sessions per week can significantly improve stress levels, sleep, and overall energy.

One important note: avoid hot yoga, especially in the three months before conception. The elevated room temperature can increase scrotal temperature and negatively affect sperm quality. Stick with regular yoga practices to gain the benefits without this risk.

Raul Pastrana

Okay, I know I've given you a lot of ideas to bring more movement into your week, but I don't want you to feel overwhelmed. You don't need to do everything at once. Even choosing one or two strategies that feel realistic for you, such as adding an extra gym session, going for regular walks, or taking up an activity you enjoy, can make a real difference.

The most important thing is consistency. Moving your body regularly supports a healthy weight, balances your hormones, reduces stress, and creates the right environment for better sperm health. For some of you, that might mean structured workouts, and for others it could be hiking in nature, cycling on weekends, or simply taking a walk after lunch. There is no single "right way" to do it. What matters is finding movement that fits your lifestyle and keeps you active over the long term.

<u>Overtraining: more common than you think</u>

When I meet a new patient, one of the first things I ask about is their physical activity. I'm always pleased to hear when exercise is part of their routine. But like many things in life, too much of a good thing can backfire.

Social media hasn't helped. Every day, we are bombarded with images of "perfect" physiques, usually paired with a product or program that promises the same results if you just train hard enough. The reality is that many of these bodies are unattainable for the average person without extreme effort, performance-enhancing drugs, or both. This constant exposure can create pressure, leading people to push themselves beyond what their bodies can recover from, convinced that more is always better.

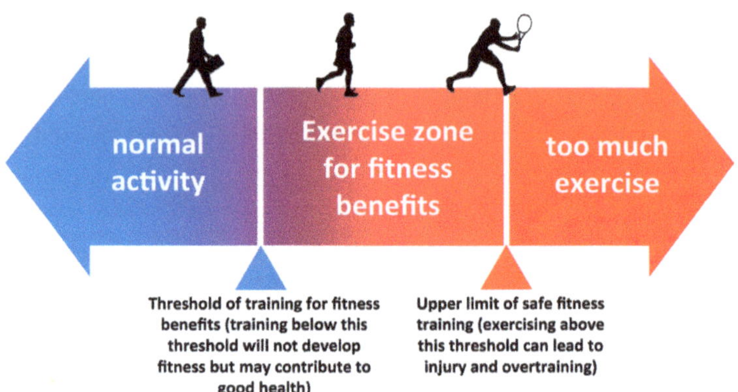

Let me be clear: I'm not here to demonise personal trainers or influencers. Most genuinely want to help their clients. But in the context of fertility, the advice to train harder, longer, and more intensely is not always the best path. Exercise is a form of stress on the body. When you recover well, that stress makes you stronger. Without proper recovery, training becomes harmful rather than helpful.

Recovery depends on many factors: training intensity and frequency, sleep quality, hydration, nutrition, hormonal health, age, baseline fitness, alcohol intake, mental well-being, and more. These factors together decide how much exercise your body can handle and adapt to. Add daily stressors from work, family, or financial pressure, and it becomes clear why some people drift into overtraining without even realising it.

The consequences tend to appear gradually: constant fatigue, irritability, poor sleep, frequent colds, slower recovery from illness, or hitting a performance plateau. Crucially for fertility, overtraining also disrupts testicular function. Research and clinical experience both show links with reduced libido, sexual dysfunction, lowered testosterone, poor semen parameters, and increased DNA fragmentation. In other words, training too hard without enough recovery doesn't just affect your muscles; it affects your sperm.

Bulking and cutting

Most gym-goers are familiar with the idea of alternating between two phases to improve body composition. Bulking involves consuming more calories than the body requires in order to build muscle mass. During this phase, it is also normal to gain some fat. This is usually followed by a cutting phase, where calorie intake is reduced to create a deficit, with the goal of losing fat while maintaining as much muscle mass as possible. Such a great theory, what could go wrong?

Sperm health and male fertility can be hugely affected by these two processes. Let's start with the most obvious one.

Cutting

When done correctly, for a short period of time and without reducing calories too aggressively, the body can usually maintain hormonal and testicular function. However, extended periods of cutting with severe caloric restriction make it difficult for the body to meet the energy and nutrient demands required for optimal testosterone production, nutrient balance, and spermatogenesis.

From an evolutionary perspective, when the body doesn't receive enough nutrients and calories over time, it shifts into a conservation state, prioritising survival functions over reproduction. In other words, the stress from calorie deprivation disrupts communication between the brain and the testes.

> Long periods of cutting = High levels of stress = Reduction in LH and FSH

This stress particularly affects LH. Without enough LH, the testes are not sufficiently stimulated to produce testosterone. In medical terms, this is called *secondary hypogonadism.*

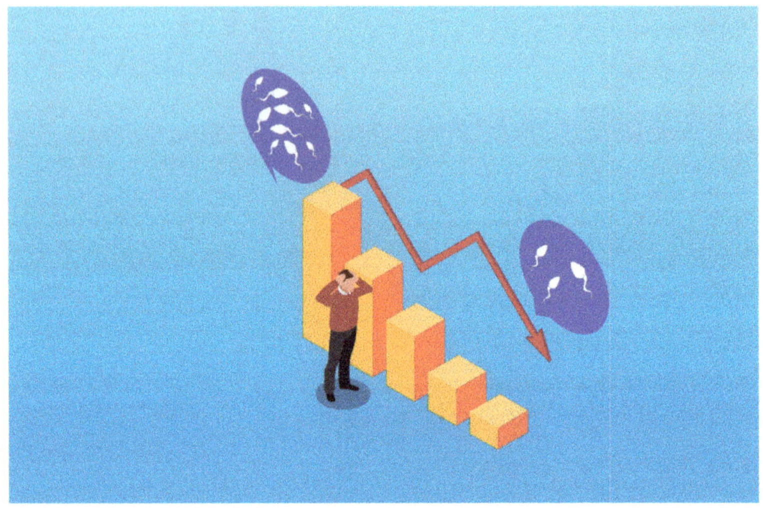

Additionally, restrictive diets can create deficiencies in key nutrients such as zinc, selenium, folate, and essential fatty acids, all of which, as we have seen in previous chapters, are critical for sperm motility, count, and DNA integrity. One could argue that supplementation can bypass this problem, and to an extent, that is correct. But cutting diets often involves a significant drop in carbohydrate intake, and this alone can trigger the hormonal changes we have discussed earlier. Supplements will not solve this issue.

I have seen this pattern many times in my practice over the years: poor semen and testosterone results caused by excessive calorie restriction. The point at which restriction becomes harmful varies from person to person, depending on their capacity to tolerate stress. Some patients can sustain high levels of stress while maintaining hormonal balance, while others see their testosterone and sperm function decline with only small changes in calorie intake.

This brings us back to a key principle: the perfect diet does not exist. We all have different bodies, strengths, and vulnerabilities. Just because a particular approach works for someone you know or follow on social media, it doesn't mean it will work for you.

Bulking

You might assume that if eating fewer calories can harm spermatogenesis and hormonal balance, eating more should help. But it's not that simple.

Eating less than your body needs is a form of stress. In the same way, consistently eating more than your body requires can also create stress. Excessive food intake, like dirty bulking (eating lots of extra calories from any kind of food, even unhealthy ones, to gain weight and muscle quickly), can overload the digestive system and lead to bloating, indigestion, and gut dysbiosis (imbalance between healthy and harmful bacteria in the gut).

Chronic overeating can cause insulin resistance, oxidative stress, and systemic inflammation. It also disrupts hunger and fullness hormones (leptin and ghrelin), which ultimately impacts testosterone levels and testicular function.

To be clear. I am not saying you should never bulk or cut. When done properly, at the right pace and for an appropriate duration, these strategies can help improve your muscle-to-fat ratio. However, if you are trying to conceive, it is best to avoid extremes of either calorie surplus or deficit.

The 3-month rule

During the three months before conception, as long as your body fat percentage is not very high or very low, the focus should be on meeting your body's energy demands while maintaining a moderate exercise routine. By doing this, you are doing your part to ensure optimal fertility and health outcomes for yourself, your partner, and your future child.

Stress management

As we've seen, stress doesn't only come from food or training. Emotional, mental, and occupational stressors can profoundly disrupt hormones and sperm health. I've observed these many times in my practice. Patients who "do everything right" with diet and exercise, yet ongoing stress keeps their hormones out of balance and their sperm parameters underperforming.

There are thousands of stress management strategies out there. I'm only going to mention a handful; practical tools that I've seen work both in research and with patients. The truth is, you don't need to try all of them. You just need to find the one (or two) that resonate with you and that you can practice consistently. Stress management isn't a one-off fix; it's a lifelong skill that we're all constantly learning and refining.

Breathwork

I'll start with breathwork because it's something I practise daily. Most mornings, I sit with my coffee and do ten to fifteen minutes of guided breathing. It helps regulate my nervous system for the rest of the day.

Meditation never fully clicked for me; it felt too abstract. Breathing, on the other hand, gives me something tangible to focus on, the rhythm of air moving in and out. It makes it easier to quiet the mind. Scientifically, breathwork activates the parasympathetic nervous system (the 'rest and digest' mode), lowers cortisol, and supports hormonal balance. Studies show that even five to ten minutes daily can reduce perceived stress, improve cardiovascular function, and benefit reproductive health.

If you've never tried it, start simple: find a YouTube channel or an app you like, and commit to ten minutes in the morning.

Cold exposure (short bursts)

We've already spoken about the importance of keeping scrotal temperature under control, but cold exposure also deserves a mention here. Finishing your shower with thirty to sixty seconds of cold water trains your nervous system to handle stress better, reduces inflammation, and boosts circulation. Personally, I find this particularly helpful in the winter months to strengthen the immune system and reduce the risk of getting sick.

When it comes to sperm health, finishing your shower with a short burst of cold water can make a real difference. That cold shock stimulates testosterone production, boosts metabolism, and sends oxygen-rich blood flowing through the body, including the testes, creating the ideal environment for hormone balance and sperm development. It might feel uncomfortable at first, but your body adapts quickly, and the benefits are worth it.

This practice can be especially valuable in the three months leading up to conception, when sperm are maturing and most sensitive to your daily habits. Even a simple thirty to sixty second cold rinse can support a healthier environment for sperm during this crucial window.

Walking outdoors and being in nature

Earlier in this book, we spoke about aiming for 10,000 steps a day. Beyond the physical benefits, walking outdoors is one of the most underrated ways to manage stress. It lowers cortisol, improves insulin sensitivity, and helps reset your nervous system after long hours of work or screen time.

If you can accumulate those steps in natural light, the benefits increase. Nature has a calming effect on the brain, helping to balance mood and hormones. Even a weekend hike can work wonders, especially after a stressful week. Time outside allows you to disconnect, recharge, and return to daily life with more clarity.

On a personal note, this is something I try to do daily with my dog. After a few hours in front of the computer, I take her for a 30–40-minute walk in the park. I leave my phone behind as often as possible (unless I need it for an important call). That time away from screens allows my brain to fully switch off, and often, when I return to work, I suddenly see solutions to problems I couldn't figure out before.

Ejaculation frequency

Ejaculation is not just about fertility. From an evolutionary perspective, it has also been a form of stress management for men. The act itself releases tension, helps regulate hormones, and resets the nervous system. But when we talk about sperm health specifically, ejaculation has an even deeper role to play.

Regular ejaculation, ideally every 2 to 3 days, is essential for maintaining healthy sperm parameters and supporting fertility. When ejaculation happens too infrequently, sperm can build up in the epididymis. Over time, these older sperm are exposed to oxidative stress, making them more prone to DNA fragmentation, reduced motility, and abnormal morphology. On the other hand, ejaculating regularly clears out older sperm and encourages the production of fresher, healthier ones.

Research backs this up. Studies have shown that those who abstained for more than 5 to 7 days often had higher semen volume but lower motility and morphology. In contrast, males who ejaculated every 2 to 3 days tended to show better overall motility, lower DNA fragmentation, and healthier sperm quality. Regular ejaculation also helps reduce inflammation and oxidative stress in the reproductive tract, creating a more supportive environment for sperm development.

In short, if you are trying to conceive or planning to freeze sperm for assisted reproductive techniques, being consistent with ejaculation every 2 to 3 days during the three months before conception or sperm banking can make a real difference in sperm quality.

A final note about stress management

The expectation here is not that you meditate an hour a day, take cold showers, practise breathwork, *and* walk 10,000 steps in nature, all at once. That's not realistic. The point is to find one practice that helps bring your nervous system into a calmer state, so your body can recover at night, you can feel better during the day, and your sperm quality can improve.

What works for you will be highly personal. I've had patients tell me that listening to heavy rock on the drive home from work is what relaxes them. Honestly, that's something I could never do to unwind, but hey, if it works for them, it works.

Stress management is less about "doing it perfectly" and more about experimenting, finding your thing, and practising it consistently. Your sperm and your whole body will thank you for it.

Sleep

In today's world, where overstimulation is the norm, sleep is often one of the first things to suffer. Both quality and quantity can be easily disrupted. Countless books are promising the "secret" to perfect sleep, but before trying the latest trend, I think it's better to start with a simple question: *why am I not sleeping well?*

The answer to that question can give you the best clues. Is there too much caffeine during the day? Scrolling on your phone late into the night, keeping your brain wired and alert? Eating heavy meals too close to bedtime, forcing your body to focus on digestion instead of rest? Once you've identified what's most relevant for you, you can begin making changes that actually matter.

Even though the ultimate goal of this book is to improve sperm quality, better sleep will improve far more than that. You'll notice higher energy, more stable moods (which means better relationships), sharper concentration, and an overall boost in wellbeing.

I'm not a "sleep expert," but poor sleep is one of the most common issues I see in my patients. From clinical experience, I've found some simple, practical foundations that make a real difference for most men:

- Consistency matters. Go to bed and wake up at the same time every day, weekends included. This trains your circadian rhythm, so your cortisol naturally tapers off at night, allowing for deeper, more restorative sleep.

- Watch your screen diet. Yes, blue light disrupts your sleep cycle, but it's not just about the light; it's about the content. If you spend hours watching violent news clips or endless social media arguments, your nervous system will stay in "fight-or-flight" mode. Even if you log off an hour before bed, your brain won't switch off easily. Think about your total daily screen exposure, not just the last hour.

- Supplement smartly. For males who need extra support, I often use a combination of L-theanine (200–400 mg), magnesium glycinate (200–400 mg), and glycine (2–3 g) to help calm the nervous system and prepare the body for rest. If you've tried this and it doesn't work for you, we have many other supplements and herbal interventions that can help.

And here's the bottom line: you may believe you "function fine" on 5 or 6 hours of sleep, but the science says otherwise. Chronic sleep deprivation (less than 7 hours per night) is consistently linked to reduced testosterone production and impaired spermatogenesis. Your body and your sperm notice the difference, even if you don't.

Alcohol: yes, it requires a special mention

Alcohol is deeply embedded in our culture. We use it to celebrate, to relax with friends, and to make a meal feel special. I know this can be a sensitive topic, and I'm not writing to shame anyone or to tell you that you must quit forever. I enjoy drinking too. My goal is to give you the evidence we now have, so you can make an informed decision, especially if you're planning to become a parent.

The reality is that alcohol has a direct impact on sperm health. Science has shown this repeatedly. Here are three key studies that illustrate the point:

1. In Denmark, researchers studied over 1,200 young males (aged 18–28 years). They found that drinking more than five drinks per week was already linked with lower sperm concentration, total sperm count, and poorer sperm shape. The pattern was dose-dependent. The more alcohol consumed, the worse the results. For example, those drinking over 25 drinks per week had dramatically lower sperm quality across every parameter compared to light drinkers. And here's what matters most: these findings were seen in relatively young men, a group that naturally has greater protection against oxidative stress and cellular damage. It is therefore only logical to expect that the same alcohol intake would have an even more damaging impact in males over 30, where natural resilience to oxidative damage declines.

2. Another study, this time in males undergoing fertility treatment, showed that even a small amount of alcohol made a measurable

difference. Those who drank seven standard drinks per week, roughly one per day, had a 9% lower chance of achieving a live birth compared to those who didn't drink at all. In other words, even moderate alcohol use can reduce IVF success rates.

3. Another study in China involving 776 males with fertility issues found the same trend. Regular drinkers had lower sperm counts and smaller testicles compared to non-drinkers. Heavy drinkers were more than three times as likely to have an abnormal sperm count. This highlights that alcohol can directly impair sperm health, especially in males already having trouble conceiving.

Together, these studies show that alcohol affects fertility in a dose-dependent way. Even small amounts matter, and heavier drinking has real consequences.

These aren't numbers. They're a wakeup call.

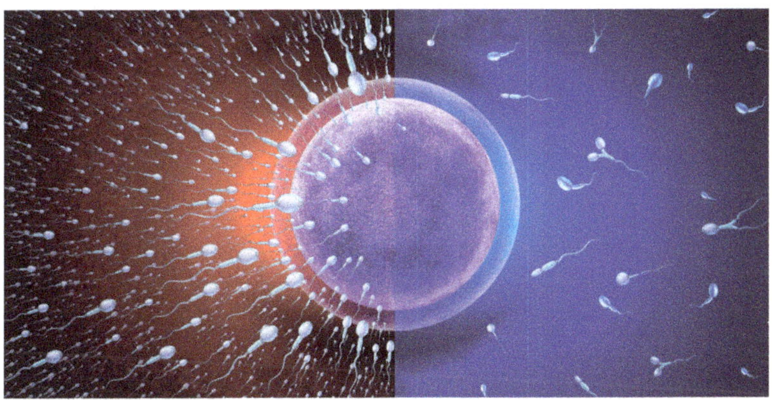

Alcohol also disrupts sperm health through hormones. It suppresses testosterone, the key hormone responsible for sperm production. Lower testosterone doesn't just mean fewer sperm; it can affect libido, energy, and mood. A review published in *Frontiers in Endocrinology* found that alcohol use is consistently associated with lower testosterone and impaired sperm parameters, making the likelihood of conception much lower. Clinically, this often shows up as males who feel tired, have low libido, and struggle to perform sexually, all before we even get to the fertility challenges.

I want to be clear. How much or how little you drink is entirely your personal choice. I never tell patients they must quit alcohol completely. If you're looking to make changes in the months leading up to conception, simply reducing your intake can already make a meaningful difference. Having an occasional drink with friends is not the end of the world. What matters most is being mindful, because protecting your sperm during this window can have an impact on the health of your future family.

There is one important exception: if you're preparing for IVF, ICSI, or planning to freeze sperm, I recommend avoiding alcohol completely for at least two weeks before the collection. The final two weeks of sperm development are crucial because this is when sperm undergo the last stages of maturation and acquire the ability to swim and carry intact DNA. Alcohol during this window can increase oxidative stress and DNA damage, directly reducing the quality of the sperm used for fertilisation, sperm that may be used to fertilise eggs your partner may have gone through months of hormones and procedures to retrieve. Avoiding alcohol in this window gives your embryos the best possible start.

I understand that making lifestyle changes can feel challenging, especially when habits are tied to your social life, routines, or ways of coping with stress. You don't have to navigate those adjustments alone. Book a consultation using the link below if you'd like personalised support to identify the most appropriate tests, better understand your results, and create a realistic, sustainable plan to improve your outcomes.

Make your booking at:

Chapter 8

Obesity & overweight: the biggest sperm killer

Carrying extra body fat is one of the most significant factors affecting fertility worldwide. Earlier, we discussed how sperm quality and quantity have been declining over the past few decades, and how this drop has accelerated since the 2000s. At the same time, another trend has been rising; more males are carrying excess weight.

Back in the 1980s, just under half of Australian males were considered overweight or obese. By the year 2000, that number had climbed to about 60%. In 2023, it's closer to 71%. That means almost 7 out of 10 male Australians are dealing with weight concerns. This isn't about looks or body image; it's about health, and it's very much about fertility.

So how do you know where you sit? A simple tool that doctors use is the Body Mass Index (BMI). You calculate it by dividing your weight (in kilograms) by your height (in meters) squared:

$$BMI = weight\ (kg) \div height\ (m)^2$$

For example, if you weigh 75kg and are 1.83m tall:
$$75 \div (1.83 \times 1.83) = 22.4$$

That result falls in the "healthy" range.

BMI Classifications Below 20: underweight

- 20 to 25: healthy range

- 25 to 30: overweight

- Over 30: obese

Now, BMI isn't perfect. It doesn't distinguish between muscle mass or body composition, so don't treat it as the ultimate verdict on your health. But it's a useful starting point. If your BMI places you in the overweight or obese range, don't see it as a judgment; it's simply information. What matters is knowing that excess weight (and in some cases, being underweight) can affect your hormones, sperm quality, and fertility outcomes.

If your BMI is higher than 25

It is absolutely possible to have a BMI over 25 and be extremely healthy and fit, as muscle weighs more than fat. If your BMI is over 25 due to the amount of muscle you carry, the following recommendations don't apply to you.

Being overweight or obese plays a huge factor in metabolic, hormonal and sperm health. Higher BMI (when not related to high muscle mass) is associated with reductions in semen volume, total sperm count, and total motile sperm count. Additionally, overweight and obese males have been found to have lower sperm count compared to those with a healthy BMI (20 to 25). The decline in these parameters is more pronounced the higher the BMI.

The bottom line here is, if you are trying to conceive and your BMI is high because you are carrying too much weight, especially around the belly area, reducing your BMI by focusing on improving your diet in combination with exercise can significantly increase your sperm health and fertility outcomes.

If you are underweight - BMI lower than 20

This is less common, but I do see it, and it can absolutely affect fertility. When the body is under-fuelled, it has a much lower tolerance to stress. That means things that would normally be fine, like a workout, a busy day at work, or even a poor night of sleep, can hit a lot harder. Instead of adapting and recovering, the body interprets it as overload. In response, cortisol (the main stress hormone) rises, and the brain turns down the signals (like LH) that tell your testes to make testosterone. With less testosterone, sperm maturation slows down. In other words, if you're under-eating, your body doesn't feel safe enough to prioritise fertility.

If this is you, the first step is to follow the nutrition principles we talked about earlier. Getting enough calories, protein, and healthy fats is essential to give your body the building blocks it needs. On top of that, strength training two to three times a week, plus aiming for no more than 10,000 steps a day, is a great starting point to build muscle and support hormone balance.

But here's the key: start slow. If your body hasn't been well-nourished, hitting the gym too hard can backfire. Pushing it with heavy workouts or loads of cardio can feel like stress to the body, which only makes the problem worse by lowering testosterone and sperm production even more. That's why long-distance running or cycling aren't the best choices here; they tend to keep cortisol levels high, and that's the last thing we want when trying to boost sperm health.

If you are on a healthy BMI higher than 20 and lower than 25

Being in this range doesn't mean there's no room to optimise. Body composition still matters. Having enough muscle mass, good circulation, and balanced hormones are all key pieces of the fertility puzzle.

When I work with males in this group, the first thing I ask about is their current activity routine. Sometimes the answer is, "I go for a couple of runs a week but never touch weights." Other times it's, "I lift five times a week but haven't done cardio in years." And then there are those who are already pushing themselves really hard in the gym, training six or seven days a week without enough recovery. Everyone's starting point is different, and the key is balance. Some need more cardio, some need more strength training, and others actually need to pull back a little and focus on rest.

If you're already consistent with exercise but still end up with a poor semen analysis, that's when I suggest digging deeper with a health professional. Exercise is just one part of the bigger picture, and sometimes it's nutrition, stress, sleep, or other hidden factors that play a bigger role in sperm health.

Chapter 9

When perfect is too perfect

Nutritional advice is everywhere, especially online. Scroll through social media platforms, and you'll find countless 'miracle diets'. The marketing is often clever, filled with before-and-after photos and stories of people who "transformed" their bodies by following a specific plan. The message is usually the same: if it worked for them, it will work for you.

Here's the thing: giving nutrition advice is not as simple as copying and pasting a plan. To do it safely and effectively, you need proper education and qualifications. While some personal trainers and coaches do have this training, many do not. Even when the advice comes from a well-meaning place, the one-size-fits-all approach fails when it comes to fertility and hormone health.

Your genetics, stress levels, digestion, intolerances, and overall lifestyle all influence how your body responds to food and exercise. I've seen many patients come to me after following strict diets that were sold to them as the "perfect plan." At first, these diets often do exactly what they promise: the weight comes off, body fat drops, and they feel like they're making progress.

But a few months in, the story often changes. When calories or entire food groups are cut too aggressively, the body starts sensing this as stress. Cortisol rises, testosterone production falls, and sperm quality declines. What started as a great strategy for fat loss turns into fatigue, low libido, and fertility struggles.

This is why individualisation is so important. A diet that works wonders for one person might completely derail another, especially when hormones and reproductive health are on the line.

I will illustrate what I mean with a case study

Case of Study: Andy 32 years old

Andy and his partner Amy had been trying to conceive for over 9 months. His semen analysis showed very low sperm count, poor morphology, and low motility. This was a real surprise to him because Andy was a healthy young male with no pre-existing medical conditions.

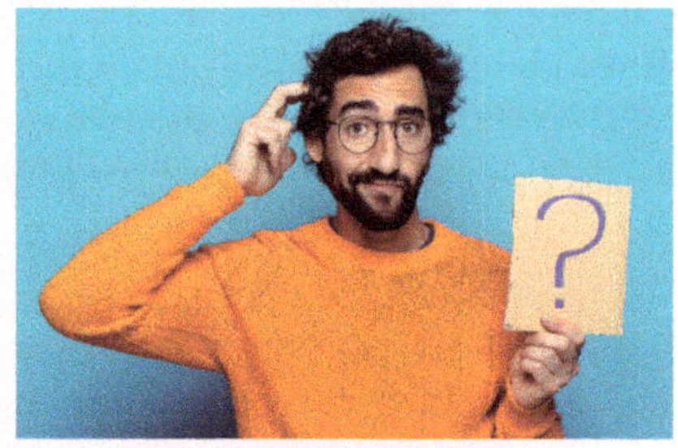

• No alcohol, smoking, or history of substance abuse.

• Fitness enthusiast: 5 gym workouts per week.

• Followed a "very healthy diet".

• Healthy BMI.

• Other than his semen analysis, his blood test looked "normal" (though hormones were tested at first).

When I asked more questions about his diet, the issue started to become clear. Andy had been eating a very low-carbohydrate diet as part of a "shredding phase" in his gym program. His goal was to reduce body fat while maintaining muscle mass. The diet had been given to him by a Personal Trainer with a strong reputation for body transformations.

Given all these factors, I started to suspect his diet was affecting his hormonal health and testicular function. I asked Andy to do a hormone blood panel, and these were some of the results:

Parameter	Andy's results	Optimal reference range
LH (Luteinizing Hormone)	1 IU/L	3 to 6/8 IU/L
FSH (Follicle Stimulating Hormone)	3 IU/L	2 to 4/6 IU/L
Total Testosterone	7.5 nmol/L	>15 -20 nmol/L
Oestrogen	45 pmol/L	50 to 120 pmol/L
Free Testosterone	118	

From the results, it was clear that his brain wasn't sending enough signals (LH and FSH) to the testes to produce testosterone and sperm.

To understand why this happens, it helps to look at how the human body has adapted over thousands of years. In times when food, especially carbohydrates, was scarce, the body had to prioritise survival over reproduction. Energy was conserved for vital functions like brain activity and movement, not for creating new life. Reproduction simply wasn't a priority if survival was at stake.

Now, fast forward to modern times. Andy wasn't starving, but his body interpreted his very low-carb diet and high training load as a signal that resources were scarce. His stress hormones, like cortisol increased, while LH and FSH dropped. The result? Low testosterone and poor sperm production. In other words, his body was saying, "This isn't the right time to reproduce, focus on survival instead."

The treatment plan for Andy was simple. He needed to increase his carbohydrate intake and slightly reduce his exercise volume while we worked on balancing his hormones. I also prescribed specific nutritional supplements and herbal compounds to improve his resilience to stress and speed up recovery. Three months later, his LH and FSH had returned to healthy ranges, and his free testosterone had doubled. By six months, Andy and Amy conceived naturally.

Why were Andy's hormones negatively affected by a diet which was so beneficial for many others?

Because we are all different. Each person has a unique exercise tolerance, the amount of physical activity our body can handle before it starts causing more harm than good. The same principle applies to carbohydrates. Some thrive on a lower-carb diet and may even need to limit foods like bread, rice, or potatoes due to factors such as a family history of diabetes. Others, however, feel and perform their best with more carbohydrates in their diet to support energy levels and hormonal balance.

We are all different and unique.
The perfect diet doesn't exist.

Nutritional advice to promote
optimal semen quality
and quantity should be
individualised based on clinical
history, blood parameters
and other factors.

Raul Pastrana

Chapter 10

Cold therapy: your balls' temperature matters

Your testicles sit outside the body for a reason; sperm need a slightly cooler environment than the rest of your body to develop properly. Even a small increase of just 1 to 2°C can slow sperm production, reduce motility, and increase DNA damage. The truth is, testicular temperature is one of the easiest fertility factors to overlook, yet one of the simplest to fix.

Modern life makes it harder than ever to maintain this delicate temperature balance. Sitting at a desk for eight hours a day presses the testes against the body, reducing the natural cooling gap. Tight underwear and synthetic fabrics trap heat. Laptops balanced on laps raise scrotal temperature within minutes. Add long commutes, hot showers, saunas, or even just your phone in your front pocket, and it becomes clear how many people are unintentionally heating their testicles every single day.

It takes 72 to 74 days for new sperm to fully develop, so small daily habits have a big cumulative effect. The good news? With a few simple adjustments, you can dramatically improve the environment your sperm grow.

What heats them up (negatives)

Tight underwear

Tight briefs, specially made from synthetic fabrics, hold the testes close to the body and trap heat. Over time, this can reduce sperm count, motility, and morphology.

Sitting for long periods

Extended sitting at a desk, in a car, or on a plane keeps the scrotum pressed against the body, narrowing airflow and raising temperature.

Laptops on your lap

Research shows scrotal temperature can rise within just 10 to 15 minutes of resting a laptop directly on your thighs. That extra heat quickly transfers to the testes, creating an environment that's far from ideal for sperm. The fix is simple. Use a desk or stand whenever possible. And if you do need to rest it on your lap, placing a firm pillow or cushion between your legs and the laptop creates enough distance to stop most of that heat from reaching your scrotum.

Hot tubs and saunas

Frequent or prolonged exposure to hot water or steam can cut sperm count by as much as 50%. While this effect is usually reversible, it's a serious consideration in the months leading up to conception or sperm collection.

To be crystal clear:

No hot baths or saunas if you're trying to conceive or planning to freeze sperm in the coming months.

Raul Pastrana

Phones in front pockets

Heat and electromagnetic radiation from phones stored near the testes have been linked to reduced sperm motility and increased DNA fragmentation. A simple fix is to keep your phone in a bag, back pocket, or jacket pocket.

How to cool things down (positives)

Boxers over briefs

Choosing looser, breathable cotton boxers instead of tight synthetic underwear helps keep the testes cooler and improves air circulation. When you're shopping, check the label. Look for 100% cotton or natural fabrics like bamboo. These materials allow airflow and wick moisture away from the skin.

Avoid underwear made mostly of polyester, which traps heat, reduces ventilation, and can raise scrotal temperature throughout the day.

Cold showers

Finishing your shower with a 30 to 60 second cold rinse doesn't just lower scrotal temperature and improve blood flow, it also supports healthy hormone function. Regular cold exposure has been shown to stimulate testosterone production, which is essential for sperm development. On top of that, cold showers enhance immunity by activating the body's natural defence systems and can boost metabolism, making it easier to manage weight, something that's especially helpful if weight gain has been a challenge.

Icing the testes

Applying a cold pack (wrapped in a towel) to the testes for 10 to 15 minutes can help lower scrotal temperature and reduce oxidative stress, creating a healthier environment for sperm production. Studies have shown that regular scrotal cooling improved sperm concentration and motility in males with fertility challenges, proof that this simple habit can make a measurable difference.

Ideally, aim to do this at least once a day, and if you have the time, even twice. Many men find it easiest on work from home days, when privacy and flexibility make it simple to build into their routine. **Important:** This should never be painful. Avoid direct ice-to-skin contact; always use a towel or thin layer of fabric as a barrier. Think of it as a gentle, consistent practice, not an extreme approach. Done properly, daily cooling is one of the easiest and most effective hacks for boosting sperm quality.

<u>Nighttime airflow</u>

Sleeping without underwear, or wearing loose boxers, allows the scrotum to cool overnight, a time when sperm regeneration is especially active.

<u>Movement breaks</u>

If you work a desk job, standing up and walking every 45 to 60 minutes isn't just good for your sperm; it helps your whole body. Regular breaks allow air to circulate in the scrotum, preventing heat build-up, but they also help regulate blood sugar. When you sit for hours without moving, your muscles become less responsive to insulin, making it harder to keep blood glucose stable. Short movement breaks improve insulin sensitivity, keep energy levels steady, and reduce the risk of weight gain.

Chapter 11

Environmental stressors: toxins, endocrine-disrupting chemicals (EDCs), and heavy metals

Modern life brings a lot of convenience, packaged foods, powerful cleaning products, supplements you can buy anywhere, but it also comes with high exposure to chemicals. Many of these compounds are known as endocrine-disrupting chemicals (EDCs), substances that can interfere with the way your hormones work. Add heavy metals like mercury and lead, and it becomes clear that our everyday decisions can have a huge impact on reproductive health.

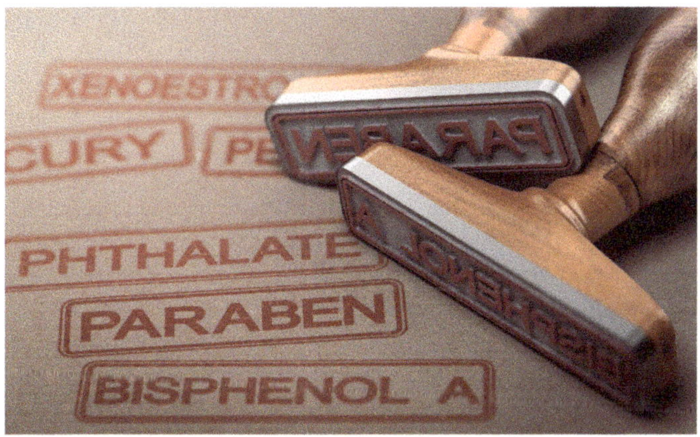

We're never going to live in a chemical-free world. Exposure is part of life. But by understanding what the biggest contributors are and making a few smarter choices, we can significantly reduce our toxic load and improve fertility outcomes.

Fish, mercury, and farmed fish

Fish is one of the best foods you can eat for fertility, but choosing the right type matters. Larger predatory fish such as sharks, swordfish, marlin, and some tuna varieties tend to have higher mercury levels. Mercury builds up in your tissues over time and can lower testosterone, damage sperm DNA, and reduce motility. Farmed fish are often exposed to higher levels of toxins such as PCBs (polychlorinated biphenyls), dioxins, and sometimes even antibiotic residues from poor farming practices. These can negatively impact both hormonal balance and sperm health.

The best fertility-friendly options are low-mercury, wild-caught fish such as salmon, sardines, anchovies, mackerel, and trout. These give you the omega-3 fatty acids your sperm needs without the heavy metal burden.

- Omega-3 Supplements can be an excellent addition to boost fertility, but quality is everything. Some of the cheaper supplements often skip proper purification, meaning they may still carry contaminants like mercury or other pollutants. If you choose to try an omega-3 supplement, make sure it has third-party testing to ensure you are taking something clean and genuinely supportive of your sperm health

Plastics and BPA

One of the biggest everyday sources of hormone disruptors is plastic. Chemicals like BPA and phthalates can leach into food and drinks, especially when plastic containers are heated in the microwave or exposed to sunlight. These chemicals mimic hormones in the body, interfering with testosterone production and sperm development.

It's worth switching to glass or stainless-steel containers, not just for cooking but also for food storage and water bottles. Plastic shows up everywhere: takeaway coffee cups (plastic lining), plastic wrap, single-use water bottles, and even some canned foods where the lining may contain BPA. The fewer of these you use, the less hormone disruption you will experience.

- Practical tip: if replacing everything at once feels overwhelming, start with the containers you use the most, your container, your water bottle, and the containers you heat meals in. Those three swaps alone can significantly lower your BPA exposure.

Cleaning products

Imagine walking into a room that's just been cleaned. You can smell it instantly, that sharp chemical "clean" scent. Some people like it, others don't. REMOVE Whether you love it or hate it, many of the chemicals behind that scent aren't great for your hormones.

Where we do have control is at home, and that's where it really matters, because it's where we spend most of our time. Many everyday cleaning products like sprays, wipes, bathroom cleaners, and multipurpose surface sprays often contain phthalates, phenols, quaternary ammonium compounds, and formaldehyde. These compounds are all known to disrupt hormones and impact sperm health.

The good news is that switching to safer alternatives has never been easier. Eco-friendly and natural cleaning products are now available in supermarkets and even more so in health food stores. If you're unsure where to start, I've included resources at the end of this chapter to help you compare brands and find options you can trust.

I feel strongly about this because the cost is usually minimal, yet the benefits to hormonal and testicular function are huge. A small swap in your cleaning cupboard can pay big dividends for your long-term fertility and health.

Personal care products

It's not just food and cleaning products. Everyday items like deodorants, shampoos, and aftershaves can also contain parabens and phthalates. These are linked to lower testosterone and poorer sperm health. Look out for products labelled "paraben-free" or "phthalate-free." Again, no need to replace your entire bathroom cabinet immediately, just start by swapping the products you use every day.

Food and pesticides

Pesticide residues on fruits and vegetables are one of the most common sources of endocrine-disrupting chemicals (EDC) exposure. As mentioned earlier, some foods are much more important to buy organic than others. Buying everything organic isn't realistic for most people, but you can still make smart choices.

Buying seasonal produce is one great option, since foods grown in season tend to be fresher, more nutrient-dense, and often carry fewer chemicals. Another option is shopping at local farmers' markets. Many smaller growers don't carry the formally certified "organic" label simply because of how expensive and time-consuming it is to get, but in my experience, they often use fewer pesticides and produce higher-quality food.

A lot of my patients also like using veggie box services. These usually cut out the supermarket middleman, which not only means fresher food arriving at your door but also allows your money to go directly to farmers. It's a practical way to buy better-quality produce while supporting small businesses at the same time.

Marketing can be misleading. Some use clever wording or loopholes in regulations to make their products look safe and natural, while still containing ingredients that aren't great for your health. Of course, there are also plenty of companies doing things properly. The point is, as consumers, we need to stay informed and take responsibility for what we bring into our homes.

If you're not sure whether the products you're using are safe, there are a few great websites where you can quickly check ingredients and see if they contain harmful chemicals.

EWG Skin Deep Database	Yuka App
https://www.ewg.org/skindeep/	https://yuka.io/en/
Use this website to check skincare, sunscreen, shampoo, deodorants etc.	You can use this app to scan barcodes of food and personal care products.
Rates each product from 1 (low hazard) to 10 (high hazard) based on chemicals, allergens, endocrine disruptors, and cancer risk	It gives you a score out of 100 based on the content of harmful ingredients, additives, pesticides and endocrine disruptors.
Think Dirty App	Chemical Maze App
https://www.thinkdirtyapp.com/	https://www.chemicalmaze.com/
You can download this app on your phone to check the quality of your personal care products and household items.	Created in Australia, focused on food additives and cosmetic ingredients.
Gives a score with clear explanations of harmful ingredients	Allow you to scan barcodes of Aussie supermarket products and see if they contain any harmful ingredients.
They offer a 7-day free trial.	This is a paying App and they don't offer free trial period.
INCIDecoder	
https://incidecoder.com/	
Great website to know if a specific ingredient is safe or has any potential risks.	

Filtering your water

If you live high up in the Swiss Alps, drinking straight from a mountain stream, this section may not apply to you. But for most of us living in major cities, we need to be a bit more careful with our water. Tap water is treated to protect us from bacteria and infectious diseases, which is important, but that doesn't mean it's free from other contaminants. Depending on where you live, trace amounts of pesticides, chlorine byproducts, pharmaceutical residues, and even heavy metals can end up in water that comes from your tap.

Individually, the levels are usually considered "safe." But here's the catch: sperm are extremely sensitive cells. Long-term, repeated exposure to these small amounts of these compounds can add up over time, contributing to oxidative stress, damaging sperm DNA, and interfering with testosterone production. Several studies have shown this pattern. For example, those living in areas with higher pesticide levels in drinking water were found to have significantly lower sperm concentration, poorer motility, and more DNA fragmentation.

The good news?

This is one of the easiest areas to take control of. A simple home water filter can dramatically reduce your exposure. Carbon filters are affordable and great at lowering chlorine, pesticides, and some pharmaceutical residues. Reverse osmosis systems go even further, removing heavy metals as well. And you don't need the fanciest setup to make a difference. Even a basic filter jug, the kind you can buy for around $50, isn't perfect, but it's a huge step in the right direction.

By choosing cleaner water, you're reducing the daily toxic load on your body. It's a small, daily habit, but over time it helps create a much healthier environment for sperm development and hormone balance.

Chapter 12

Medical considerations: varicocele, infections, diabetes and medications

Some health conditions play a much bigger role in sperm quality than people realise. Things like varicocele, infections, or metabolic conditions such as diabetes can have a direct impact on how sperm is produced and how well it functions. In my experience, too many couples get told they have "unexplained infertility" before anyone has properly ruled these factors out.

Getting the right diagnosis matters because if you know what's going on, you can take targeted action. That might mean medical treatment, or it could mean targeted lifestyle changes and supplements. Either way, identifying the underlying issue can make a significant difference.

Varicocele

Varicocele is essentially varicose veins, but instead of being in the legs, they're in the scrotum. Around 15% of males in the general population have them, and the number jumps to about 40% in those dealing with infertility. Interestingly, most varicoceles are found on the left side because of the way the veins are structured and how blood drains in that area.

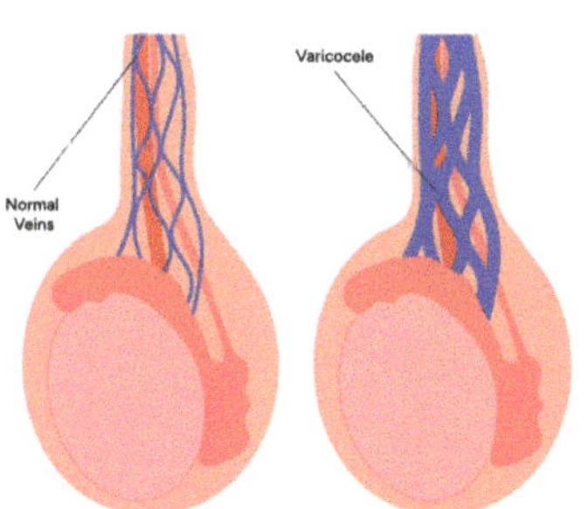

The reason varicocele can affect sperm health comes down to a few key changes it causes in the testes. Firstly, it interferes with the natural cooling system. Sperm production is very temperature sensitive and must happen at about 34–35°C, a couple of degrees cooler than the rest of the body. When the veins are enlarged, blood doesn't circulate as efficiently, and the scrotal temperature rises. Even a small increase is enough to throw sperm production off balance.

Varicoceles are also linked to higher levels of oxidative stress. This means there's an excess of reactive oxygen species (ROS) in the semen, which can damage the sperm's outer membrane, increase DNA fragmentation, and interfere with energy production in the mitochondria, all of which reduce sperm quality.

Finally, varicocele can affect hormone balance. It may impair the function of the Leydig cells, the ones responsible for producing testosterone. Since testosterone is essential for healthy sperm development and maturation, this disruption can further contribute to fertility issues.

The most common findings I have seen with varicocele patients in their semen analysis are:

- Reduce sperm concentration
- Poor progressive motility
- Abnormal morphology
- Increase DNA fragmentation

So yes, varicocele can affect every major parameter of sperm health. This is important to keep in mind because many patients with varicocele are quickly offered Assisted Reproductive Techniques (ART) like IVF or ICSI. While these technologies can help overcome some of the fertility barriers, the reality is that varicocele still lowers IVF success rates, mainly because it impacts embryo quality.

Embryologists can select the sperm that appear the healthiest under the microscope, the ones with good shape (morphology) and movement (motility). But here's the catch: they can't see what's inside the sperm. If the DNA is damaged, that won't be obvious until after the sperm has been used for fertilisation. Only then, can embryos be tested using

PGT (which we've already talked about earlier in the book) to check the quality of the combined genetic material of the embryo.

Now picture this. As a couple, you've gone through the effort of collecting eggs. Wouldn't it make sense to make sure the sperm going into the process are in the best possible shape beforehand? By improving sperm health before fertilisation, you're increasing the likelihood of a healthy pregnancy.

<u>Varicocele diagnosis</u>

Varicocele can often be detected during a physical examination by a qualified doctor, usually a urologist. They may be able to feel the enlarged veins in the scrotum, especially when you're standing up or performing a gentle "bearing down" movement (similar to straining as if lifting something heavy).

However, the most reliable way to confirm the diagnosis is with a scrotal ultrasound, which measures flow and vein size. The gold standard is finding a venous dilation greater than 2–3 mm.

It's important to emphasise that only a medical professional can diagnose varicocele. If you suspect it because of symptoms like a heavy feeling in the scrotum, visible enlarged veins, or abnormal semen results, the next step is to check in with your doctor. An accurate diagnosis offers clarity and opens the door to the right treatment options.

<u>How can you treat varicocele?</u>

From a conventional medical perspective, the management of varicocele remains a debated topic. However, growing evidence suggests that varicocelectomy (surgical repair of varicocele) can improve pregnancy rates in couples affected by male factor infertility. Research suggests it may enhance sperm concentration, motility, morphology, and DNA integrity, often reducing the number of IVF cycles required.

In clinical practice, many couples are advised to proceed directly to IVF or ICSI. This recommendation can be appropriate, particularly because improvements in semen parameters after varicocele repair may take 6 to 12 months to appear. One study reported that about 60% of patients experienced a significant improvement in at least one parameter within six months of surgery. But this also means that around 40% did not show a measurable improvement. Outcomes depend on various factors, including the severity, age, duration of infertility, and baseline sperm quality.

This is why each case requires individual consideration. For couples not under immediate time pressure to conceive, for example, when maternal age is not a limiting factor, surgical intervention can be worthwhile and potentially improve long-term fertility outcomes. However, when time is critical, proceeding with assisted reproductive techniques may be the more practical path.

Ultimately, discussing your options with your andrologist or urologist to understand the risks, benefits, and timing so you can make a decision that best fits your situation.

Natural approach to varicocele

Regardless, whether you opt for surgery or not, there are other interventions anyone with a varicocele can start doing to improve their semen health:

1. Cold therapy: 10 to 15 minutes of cold therapy in the scrotum area. We have already discussed the benefits of doing this in general for anyone wanting to improve their semen parameters. But when it comes to varicocele, it is even more important. I like to ask my patient to apply cold 2 to 3 times per day. This will help reduce scrotal temperature and improve the environment for optimal spermatogenesis.

2. Increase antioxidants to mitigate the increase of Reactive Oxygen Species associated with varicocele. I like to use antioxidant supplementation (high dosages) for a period of at least 6 months. Some of the most common ones include NAC, selenium, CoQ10 and l-carnitine.

3. Support hormonal function with herbs to promote optimal testosterone function. I like to use specific herbs depending

on the patient's needs. Tribulus, Korean Ginseng and Tongkat Ali are some of my preferred choices.

4. Support venous integrity with other herbs like Horse Chestnut and Bilberry.

I would like to emphasise, I don't recommend anyone to do all of this at once. It is always important to assess and understand the person in front of you to choose which of these many interventions and treatment options is most appropriate. What herb, what supplements, at what dosage and for how long depends on the individual.

Infections

Any major stress on the body can take a toll on sperm health, and infections are a big contributor. Whether viral, bacterial, or even fungal, infections trigger inflammation and oxidative stress. Because spermatogenesis is such a delicate process, this extra stress can easily disrupt it. One of the first questions I ask patients is, "When was the last time you were sick?" That simple detail can give important clues and help guide further testing.

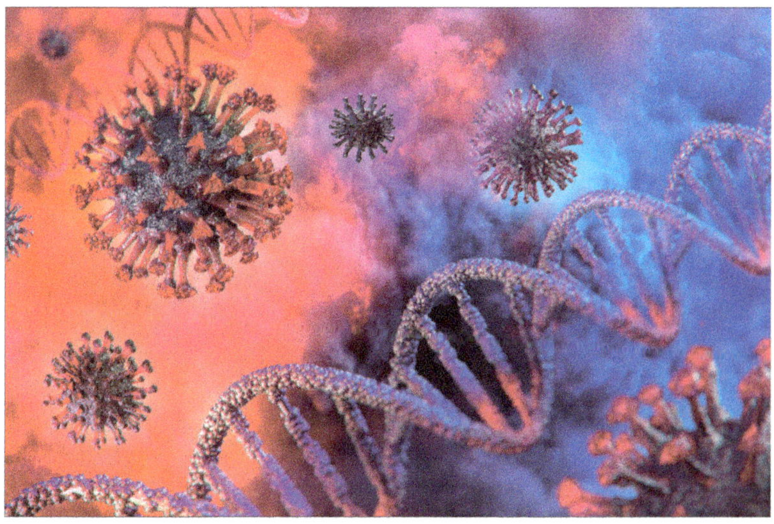

A special mention here goes to COVID-19. We now know it can negatively affect male reproductive health, not just during the infection but for months afterwards. A 2021 study found that males recovering from moderate COVID had significantly lower sperm concentration and motility. The good news is that for most men, sperm parameters tend to bounce back within 3 to 6 months, but in some cases, recovery is slower, especially if the illness was severe.

This is why I often give my patients an immune support protocol to help speed up recovery and support healthy spermatogenesis. Waiting at least three months post-infection, while supporting your body with the right nutrients and lifestyle, can make a noticeable difference in restoring sperm quality. Whether you're trying naturally or preparing for IVF, recognising and addressing the impact of recent infections is an important step.

Diabetes and insulin resistance: blood glucose control

When everything in the body is functioning well, after you eat a meal, your blood sugar rises for a short time, and then your body releases insulin. Insulin works like a key, helping glucose move from the blood stream into your cells, where it can be used for energy. Once that happens, blood sugar levels drop back to normal, and the system resets.

Problems arise when this balance is disrupted. Diabetes is the condition most people are familiar with, where blood sugar remains too high because insulin is either not being made properly (type I) or the body is not responding to it effectively (type II). High blood sugar creates inflammation and oxidative stress throughout the body, and the testes are especially vulnerable. Research has shown that those with diabetes often have poorer sperm quality, including lower motility, abnormal shape, and more DNA damage.

Most patients who already have diabetes know how important blood sugar control is for their fertility. What is often overlooked is that trouble begins long before diabetes develops. This stage is called insulin resistance. In insulin resistance, the body has to produce more insulin to achieve blood glucose control. On a standard blood test, glucose might still look normal, but the high levels of insulin could already be causing harm. Elevated insulin increases inflammation, interferes with hormone balance, reduces blood flow to the testes, and creates oxidative stress that damages sperm.

I see this all the time in clinic. Males who look fit and healthy on the outside sometimes show clear signs of insulin resistance when we run their blood work, and it is almost always connected to fertility issues. And while being overweight makes insulin resistance more likely, I often see patients with a perfectly healthy body weight who still have pre-diabetes or poor metabolic health. You cannot judge metabolic health just by appearance, which is why testing is so important.

Here is what blood tests can tell us based on standard reference values

- Fasting Insulin: Levels above 10 to 15 uIU/mL point to insulin resistance, even if glucose looks fine.

- Fasting Glucose: A reading between 5.6 and 6.9 mmol/L is considered impaired fasting glucose, or pre-diabetes.

That is the textbook definition. In my clinical practice, especially when fertility is the focus, I work with tighter targets. I like to see fasting insulin under 8 uIU/mL, ideally closer to 6. For fasting glucose, the best range is between 4.5 and 5 mmol/L. When patients reach these levels, I consistently see improvements in sperm quality, including better motility, higher counts, and less DNA fragmentation. Better control of blood glucose and insulin levels creates a healthier environment in the testes where sperm can mature properly.

One tool that has been a real breakthrough in recent years is continuous glucose monitoring, or CGM. Devices such as the Freestyle Libre stick painlessly to the back of the arm, usually near the triceps, and connect directly to your phone through an app. Instead of getting just one or two numbers from a blood test, you can see exactly how your body responds to different meals, exercise, stress, or even sleep. Many of my patients are surprised to find that foods they thought were harmless spike their glucose. Having this kind of feedback makes it much easier to adjust your lifestyle and see what truly works for your body.

Whether you use simple fasting blood tests or more advanced tools like CGMs, understanding how your body handles glucose is a powerful tool for your fertility. Good blood sugar control is not only about preventing diabetes later in life; it is about giving your sperm the optimal environment to thrive today.

Natural approach to diabetes and insulin resistance

I know I'm repeating myself here, but it's important to understand the differences between diabetes and insulin resistance, because each behaves differently and requires a different approach.

Type I diabetes is an autoimmune condition in which the pancreas stops producing insulin completely. Insulin therapy is essential; there's no alternative, and medical supervision is non-negotiable. Lifestyle habits like exercise, diet, and stress reduction can support overall health and improve sperm quality, but they cannot replace insulin.

Type II diabetes, on the other hand, is a very different story. In this case, the body can still produce some insulin, sometimes in very high amounts, but the cells don't respond to it properly. Here, lifestyle changes can make a profound difference. With the right approach, many males can reduce their reliance on insulin or medication, improve blood sugar control, and in some cases even put their diabetes into remission. Of course, this should always be done with proper medical supervision, and combining treatment with lifestyle is where I see the best outcomes.

Insulin resistance is the stage before Type II diabetes. At this stage, blood sugar on a test might still look "normal," but insulin levels are already elevated and causing silent damage. The positive news is that insulin resistance is fully reversible. I see it all the time in practice: with the right nutrition and regular movement, patients restore insulin sensitivity, reduce inflammation, and create a significantly better environment for sperm production.

What can you do in your daily life to support blood glucose control?

One of the simplest and most effective habits is walking after meals. A ten to fifteen-minute walk after eating helps muscles absorb glucose, reducing blood sugar spikes, and easing the workload on insulin. This is one of the most powerful yet underrated tools I recommend to my patients.

Diet plays a major role, too. Reducing carbohydrate load is key, especially avoiding "naked carbs," which means eating carbohydrates alone on an empty stomach. Pairing carbs with protein, fat, or fibre slows digestion and prevents large spikes in blood glucose. Over time, this makes the body more sensitive to insulin. Most males with insulin resistance also have poor carbohydrate tolerance, meaning they thrive on higher protein and healthy fats, and lower carbohydrate intake.

Building muscle is a huge factor. Muscle tissue acts as a glucose sponge. The more muscle you have, the more room your body has to store and process glucose without needing huge amounts of insulin. This is why resistance training is so important, not just for fertility, but also for long-term metabolic health.

As for general diet principles, the focus should be on whole, unprocessed foods. Think plenty of vegetables, lean proteins, healthy fats like olive oil, avocado, and nuts, and controlled portions of slow-digesting carbs such as legumes and whole grains. Avoid refined carbs, sugary drinks, and constant snacking. These habits evaluate insulin levels considerably, which is exactly what we want to avoid.

Certain supplements can support this process. There are a few nutrients and herbs that can make a big difference. Alpha-lipoic acid, chromium, herbs such as berberine, cinnamon and gymnema, to mention a few.

To be clear, if you have Type I or Type II diabetes, medication management comes first, and these natural strategies are there to support and enhance your results. But if you are at the stage of insulin resistance or pre-diabetes, *this* is the time to intervene. With the right lifestyle and nutritional support, you can completely turn things around, creating a far healthier environment for sperm production.

Chapter 13

Medications, drugs and pharmaceuticals

These days, it is very common to be taking some form of pharmaceutical medication, whether it's an antidepressant, an anti-inflammatory, cholesterol medication, and so on. That's the simple reality of modern medicine: there's usually a pill to manage each symptom or condition. The point of this chapter is not to debate whether these medications are good or bad. Many of them are essential and, in many cases, lifesaving. Without antibiotics, for example, a simple infection could still be dangerous. And for someone navigating depression, an antidepressant might be exactly what's needed to regain stability.

What I want to emphasise is something that often goes unnoticed: medications can have significant effects on spermatogenesis and on hormonal balance. Testicular function is extremely sensitive. As previously outlined, stress, diet, and toxins can influence sperm outcomes, but pharmaceuticals can also shift the body's biochemistry in ways that affect fertility. This doesn't mean you should stop taking a prescribed medication; that decision must always be made during a conversation with your doctor. The goal here is awareness. If you wish to understand how a certain medication might affect sperm, you can support your system more effectively and make informed decisions alongside your healthcare team.

Below, we'll look at some of the most common classes of medications and how they interact with male fertility.

Antidepressants / selective serotonin reuptake inhibitors (SSRIs)

SSRIs are among the most commonly prescribed medications for depression, anxiety, premature ejaculation, and certain types of pain. Well-known examples include escitalopram, fluvoxamine, paroxetine, fluoxetine, and sertraline.

In 2022, a systematic review looked at the effect of SSRIs on semen quality. The findings were consistent. After only three months of treatment, sperm concentration, sperm motility, and DNA fragmentation were negatively affected. This shows us that SSRIs can impact semen quality in the short term.

What is less clear from the scientific research is the long-term effect of using these medications for years. In my clinical practice, however, I have seen a strong correlation. Many patients who have been on SSRIs for a long time present with poor semen results. The trend I have observed is that both dosage and length of treatment matter. Higher doses and longer use often lead to more noticeable effects on sperm quality.

Here is an example. A patient I who had been on sertraline for nearly a decade, taking 150 mg daily presented with these results

Parameter		Reference ranges based on the 5th percentile	Reference ranges based on the 50th percentile
Semen Volume	4.7 ml	> 1.5ml	3.7ml
Sperm Concentration	6.4 million/ml	>15 million/ml	73 million/ml
Total Sperm Count	30.08 million	>39 million	255 million
Sperm Motility (progressive)	13%	>32%	55%
Sperm Morphology	2.6 %	> 4%	15%

His results were nowhere near the 5th percentile. And as we have already established, being close to the lower reference range doesn't mean the sperm is of good quality. A better comparison is always with the 50th percentile, which gives us a much clearer picture of what "healthy" sperm should look like.

For this patient, there were several contributing factors. We worked together on improving his nutritional status, calming his constant fight-or-flight stress response, improving both the duration and quality of his sleep, and cutting down on alcohol. At the same time, I collaborated with his GP to gradually reduce his sertraline dosage from 150 mg to 50 mg.

After eight months of this combined approach, his semen analysis results had improved dramatically:

Parameter		Reference ranges based on the 5th percentile	Reference ranges based on the 50th percentile
Semen Volume	5.9 ml	> 1.5ml	3.7ml
Sperm Concentration	29 million/ml	>15 million/ml	73 million/ml
Total Sperm Count	171 million	>39 million	255 million
Sperm Motility (progressive)	51 %	>32%	55%
Sperm Morphology	12 %	> 4%	15%

Not long after, he and his partner were able to conceive naturally. While it's true that we worked on several areas at once, diet changes, targeted supplements, and herbs, I genuinely don't believe we would have achieved this level of improvement without also reducing SSRI dosage.

This is just one example of how strongly these medications can influence testicular function. Of course, every patient's situation is unique, and for some, it may not be possible, or even safe, to reduce their dosage. That's why these decisions must always be made alongside a medical professional. Still, awareness of these effects allows us to make more informed decisions and to explore alternatives when the timing and circumstances are right.

The hair medication: 5-Alpha reductase inhibitors

Finasteride and dutasteride are the two main medications in the 5-alpha reductase inhibitor family, something you've likely heard about if you've ever looked into hair loss treatments. They work by blocking the enzyme that converts testosterone into dihydrotestosterone (DHT), the hormone responsible not just for hair loss, but also for prostate enlargement and oily skin.

I've seen plenty of patients and friends use finasteride or dutasteride with great success to slow down or even stop hair loss. It's a personal choice, there's no right or wrong here; however, it is important to be aware of the impact these medications can have on sperm health, especially if you are trying to conceive.

A 2007 study found that after one year of daily finasteride or dutasteride, there were mild but noticeable reductions in sperm count, semen volume, and motility, but these changes were mostly reversed within six months after stopping the medication. This tells us that while these medications may affect sperm, those effects are typically not permanent.

Of course, not everyone can or wants to stop these medications, especially if they're helping with urinary symptoms. But for those taking them for hair loss and hoping to conceive, it's worth having an honest conversation with your doctor. Even a temporary pause may lead to meaningful improvements in sperm quality.

Cholesterol drugs: statins

Statins are among the most prescribed medications for high cholesterol. They are often given as a first-line intervention, even though for many patients, diet and lifestyle changes could make a huge difference without the need for statins. In my opinion, this drug class is the perfect example of how modern medicine tends to reach for a pill instead of first addressing the root cause. In many cases, high cholesterol is linked to diet, weight, and sedentary lifestyle, factors that can often be improved with the right lifestyle approach.

That said, statins are sometimes needed. They save lives, especially for patients with a strong family history of genetic cholesterol issues like familial hypercholesterolemia. In those cases, the body is genetically programmed to produce excess cholesterol, and lifestyle alone is rarely enough. But for the majority of patients, there's usually more room to explore diet and exercise before committing to lifelong medication.

The most common names you might recognise are rosuvastatin (Crestor), atorvastatin (Lipitor), and simvastatin (Zocor). They work by blocking an enzyme in the liver that produces cholesterol, which helps bring down overall cholesterol levels in the blood.

When it comes to sperm health, research has shown that statins can have an impact. For example, animal studies using Rosuvastatin found a significant reduction in sperm concentration, while Simvastatin has been linked to changes in Leydig cells, the cells in the testes responsible for testosterone production. Mechanistically, this is easy to understand. Testosterone is produced from cholesterol, and when cholesterol is suppressed, the testes may struggle to produce optimal testosterone levels. In turn, this can compromise sperm quality and fertility potential.

If you're taking statins, it's important not to stop suddenly. Always speak with your doctor before making changes. What I've seen in practice is that, under medical supervision, patients who successfully improve their diet and physical activity often can reduce their statin dosage, or in some cases, discontinue the medication altogether. When it's not possible to stop medication, there are clinical interventions we employ which are able to reduce some of the negative side effects on sperm production.

Anabolic steroids & TRT

If you have ever used anabolic steroids or testosterone replacement therapy (TRT), this section is especially important for you. This isn't about shaming anyone. It's about giving you clarity on how these drugs may have affected, or may still be affecting, your sperm health. In recent years, I've seen a growing number of patients come into my clinic with fertility challenges that can be traced back to previous steroid use.

Anabolic steroid use has grown significantly over the last few decades. It's no longer limited to elite athletes. Many everyday gym-goers and bodybuilding enthusiasts are turning to these drugs in search of faster muscle growth or to achieve a leaner appearance. Some studies even suggest that in certain fitness environments, as many as one in four males (25%) report having used anabolic steroids.

Anabolic steroids are synthetic substances designed to mimic or exaggerate the effects of testosterone. When introduced into the body, they flood the system with "too much" testosterone. The brain responds by switching off its own signals to the testes, reducing or even stopping the release of LH, the hormone that tells the testes to produce testosterone. Without that stimulation, the testes begin to shrink, and sperm production slows down or even stops altogether.

MALE REPRODUCTIVE HORMONES

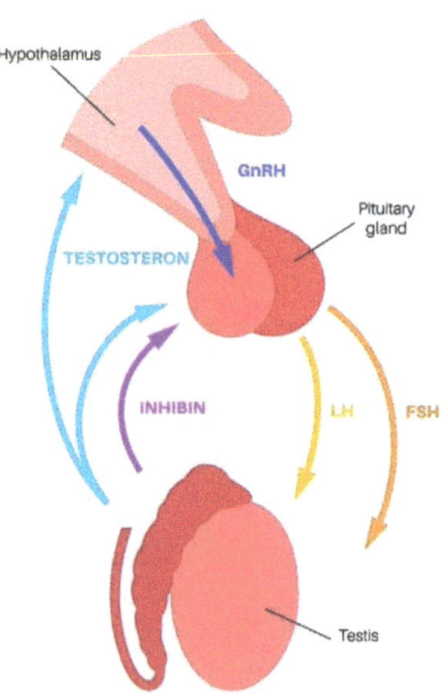

The long-term consequences of anabolic steroids can be serious. Testicular shrinkage and infertility are common outcomes when LH stimulation shuts down. Natural testosterone levels can drop sharply once steroids are stopped, sometimes for months, for years, and in a few cases, they never return to normal. Many males also experience mood swings, acne, low libido, fatigue, cardiovascular strain, liver stress, and mental health challenges that linger well after use has ended.

It's important to understand that not everyone shows obvious side effects. Some males may feel like they've managed to enjoy the benefits of steroids with minimal issues. But here's the truth: the reduction in sperm production happens whether or not you notice other symptoms. You may not see or feel the changes, but your fertility can still be impacted in a very real way.

That's why, if you've ever used anabolic steroids or TRT in the past, a thorough semen analysis is essential. This is the only way to properly assess how your sperm health has been affected and to understand what steps you may need to take for recovery. Even if you feel fine and your testosterone levels seem normal, checking your sperm quality is an essential part of protecting your fertility.

Recovery is possible in many cases, but it takes time. Since sperm production runs on a 72- to 74-day cycle, it usually takes several months before improvements can be seen in a semen analysis. Lifestyle changes, diet, and supplements all help, but the most critical factor is simply giving the testes time to re-establish their function.

In some cases, recovery can be supported with medical treatment. Endocrinologists may prescribe medications such as hCG (human chorionic gonadotropin) or clomiphene citrate. These drugs mimic the brain's natural signals, encouraging the testes to restart testosterone and sperm production. When done under medical supervision, I've seen these approaches help patients recover faster.

There's also a psychological aspect to steroid use that deserves attention. Many males begin using these drugs due to body image pressures or the desire to perform in competitive fitness environments. Social media only amplifies this by showcasing lean, muscular bodies that are often enhanced by drugs. For younger people in particular, this can create enormous pressure, and steroids may seem like the only way to keep up. The problem is that while these substances may deliver results in the short term, the long-term costs to fertility, health can be significant.

When I meet patients with poor semen results linked to previous steroid use, my role is never to judge. Some patients come in already feeling regret or shame about their past choices, while others don't feel that way at all. Both are completely valid. What matters is creating a safe space where they can be open and honest, so we can focus fully on recovery. The encouraging truth is that with time, consistent lifestyle support, and in some cases medical treatment, many males can restore their sperm health and go on to conceive naturally.

Ibuprofen

Certain pain and anti-inflammatory medications like ibuprofen are some of the most commonly used over-the-counter drugs worldwide. They are usually safe in the short term, but when it comes to male fertility, long-term or frequent use may be more harmful than most people think. These drugs can interfere with enzymes involved in hormone regulation and testicular function. For example, studies have shown that prolonged ibuprofen use may slightly lower testosterone production by disrupting the normal communication between the brain and the testes.

A recent 2025 paper published in the *European Journal of Obstetrics & Gynecology and Reproductive Biology* illustrates this effect. The study showed that males who used ibuprofen for more than 60 days per year had double the risk of receiving a clinical infertility diagnosis compared to those using paracetamol over the same period. This reinforces the idea that regular, long-term ibuprofen use may have a measurable impact on male reproductive function.

Now, this doesn't mean you need to panic if you take a couple of tablets for a headache or muscle soreness. Occasional or short-term use is generally considered safe and unlikely to have a major impact on sperm quality. The bigger concern is for patients who rely on these medications daily or for weeks at a time, whether for chronic pain, sports injuries, or inflammatory conditions.

Because it takes about three months for new sperm to fully develop, I explain to my patients that this is a key window where every choice matters. When male patients hear this, many decide on their own to cut back on unnecessary painkillers during this time. Instead of automatically reaching for ibuprofen for every mild ache, they sometimes choose to try rest, hydration, stretching, or other simple strategies first.

The point isn't about never taking a painkiller again, but about being more mindful in those three months before conception. For many patients, this small adjustment feels like an easy and practical way to support better sperm health.

Cannabis

Cannabis (or weed) is one of the most widely used recreational drugs worldwide. In Australia, it was legalised for medicinal and scientific purposes in 2016. To obtain a prescription, you must go through an Authorised Prescriber Doctor. Medicinal cannabis is usually prescribed for conditions such as chronic pain, insomnia, anxiety, multiple sclerosis, epilepsy, or chemotherapy-induced nausea.

Since then, the medicinal cannabis industry in Australia has grown massively. Increasing numbers of patients are getting access to oils, tinctures, dry flower, gummies, edibles, and sprays, often in different combinations of THC and CBD depending on their condition. Personally, I think this has been a significant step in the right direction. Previously, many people were buying cannabis illegally from unregulated sources, where quality and contamination posed a higher risk. Now, there's a safe and regulated way to access it. Clinically, I've seen plenty of patients benefit by managing their pain, anxiety, or improving their sleep with the right prescription.

That said, when it comes to male fertility, cannabis use needs careful consideration. Multiple studies have shown that regular cannabis use can lower sperm count, reduce motility, cause abnormal morphology, and increase DNA fragmentation. Cannabinoids like

THC interact with the endocannabinoid system, which plays a vital role in testosterone balance and spermatogenesis. Some research even shows that heavy use can lower testosterone by suppressing LH, the hormone that stimulates the testes to make it. Less testosterone means less stimulation for sperm maturation.

One thing that often gets overlooked is that frequency and dosage matter. Having the occasional puff or using cannabis lightly doesn't carry the same risk as heavy or frequent use. But in patients who are using it frequently, especially in higher doses, the impact on sperm quality is much more obvious. I see this a lot in clinic: the heavier the use, the worse the semen results tend to be.

Perhaps the biggest concern is DNA fragmentation. We've already discussed how higher DNA damage in sperm leads to poor embryo quality, lower implantation rates, and a higher risk of miscarriage. This is especially relevant for couples going through IVF or ICSI, because even though the lab can select sperm with better motility and morphology, they can't see DNA damage inside the sperm.

Because the sperm take about 72 days to fully develop, I always recommend my patient to check with their medical provider for possible alternatives to cannabis for the three months before conception. This gives the body time to produce a new batch of sperm with improved quality, assuming other lifestyle factors are also being addressed.

CBD vs THC

THC is the main psychoactive compound in cannabis, the one that gives the "high." CBD, on the other hand, is non-psychoactive and is often used more for its calming or pain-relieving effects. When it comes to fertility, studies have consistently shown that regular THC use is linked to negative outcomes for male reproductive health. Sperm count, motility, morphology, and DNA integrity can all be affected.

CBD hasn't been studied as much, but what we do know suggests that low to moderate doses of CBD appear to be relatively safe when it comes to sperm health. Although extremely high dosages may affect sperm function. Again, frequency and dosage matter.

I don't believe in a one-size-fits-all approach where everyone who is trying to conceive should stop cannabis completely. For some, medicinal cannabis may be the only thing that helps manage chronic pain, anxiety, depression, or sleep issues. But if cannabis use is mainly recreational, reducing or pausing during the preconception period could give your sperm and your future baby a better start.

Chapter 14

Supplementation: Does it work?

Do I need supplementation if my diet is healthy?

This is a question that has sparked endless debate, but here is the honest answer: Yes, *I do believe in supplementation*, especially when it comes to improving male fertility. This is not just an opinion. Countless scientific studies show how many nutrients, vitamins and compounds can improve sperm health.

One of the biggest reasons why supplementation is often necessary is simply the world we live in today. The food we buy at supermarkets is often lacking vitamins, minerals, and other key nutrients. Soil depletion, large-scale farming practices, and long transport chains all mean that what you see on your plate may not carry the same nutritional value it once did. For example, spinach can lose up to 90 percent of its vitamin C content within a few days of being harvested, long before it reaches your plate. Similarly, unripe fruits and vegetables picked for shipping often never reach their full nutrient potential, and even whole grains lose a significant portion of their B vitamin content during standard processing and packaging.

This means that even if you are following what appears to be a balanced, healthy diet, it is still possible to develop nutritional deficiencies. This is where supplementation becomes a powerful tool to bridge the gap and give the body what it needs to function at its best.

Repeatedly in my practice, I have seen how the right vitamins, minerals, herbs, and nutrients at the right dosage can completely shift someone's semen analysis. Many of my patients have improved sperm count, motility, morphology, and even DNA integrity by combining a targeted supplement strategy with the right lifestyle changes.

But here is the catch. This is not how most people use supplements. The reality is that the supplement industry has exploded over the last decade, and with it, endless promises of 'higher testosterone', 'higher libido', 'better erections', 'more energy', and 'anti-ageing' effects. The problem is that most of these formulas are designed for the masses, with one formula and one dose for everyone. And that is *not* how the human body works.

<u>So how do you make sense of it all? Let's break it down.</u>

1. <u>What are you actually treating?</u>

If you're going to spend money on a supplement, first ask yourself: what am I trying to fix? The reason your sperm isn't performing well will not be the same as the next person's. That's why I always start with a blood test and semen analysis. Without knowing whether the problem is oxidative stress, nutrient deficiency, hormonal imbalance, or something else, you're basically throwing darts in the dark.

2. <u>Dosage: usually not enough</u>

This is probably the number one reason so many supplements don't work. A lot of brands sell vitamins, minerals, and herbs that are severely underdosed. For fertility-related supplements, you generally need a minimum of 3 months of consistent use to see meaningful results (sometimes longer, depending on your baseline levels). But if you're taking a "fertility booster" with 30mg of CoQ10 when research shows you need 150–300mg, you're simply wasting your time and money.

On the flip side, dosage can also go the other way. Too much of a good thing can cause problems, and in rare cases even toxicity. Over the last year, for example, there's been more awareness around vitamin B6 toxicity, which can occur with very high dosages and lead to nerve damage. While these cases are uncommon, they're a good reminder that more is not always better. This is exactly why dosage matters so much; it must be enough to be effective, but not so much that it becomes harmful.

3. <u>Quality matters</u>

The market is absolutely flooded with supplement companies, each promising "revolutionary" or "clinically proven" formulas. Some may be effective, but plenty are poor in quality. Contaminants, fillers, or weak raw ingredients can make a huge difference to whether the supplement actually works. Herbs are especially sensitive to sourcing. Soil quality, harvesting, processing and storage influence potency. An herb grown in poor soil or processed badly will never deliver the same therapeutic effect as one sourced carefully.

And the marketing doesn't help, the label will usually be shouting exactly what you want to hear in big bold letters: "testosterone booster," "fertility enhancer," "clinically proven results." But what really matters is the ingredient list and the actual quantities. That's where you'll see whether the supplement is underdosed, overdosed, or uses cheap fillers instead of high-quality compounds. If you don't look past the label, it's very easy to be misled.

4. <u>Not a magic solution</u>

In the clinic, I rarely separate lifestyle changes from supplements. For example, if stress and poor sleep are an issue, I might pair magnesium and calming herbs alongside lifestyle strategies to reduce that fight-or-flight response. The synergy is what makes the difference. Think of supplements as one piece of the puzzle; they work best when combined with the bigger lifestyle picture rather than being treated as a 'magic fix'.

5. <u>Not any supplement for anyone</u>

This is probably the biggest misconception pushed by big brands. The idea that "this pill will improve semen quality in all men" is simply not true. The truth is that your genetic makeup, metabolism, hormone balance, and lifestyle all influence what you actually need. That's why what worked wonders for your friend may do nothing for you or even make things worse.

The takeaway is this. Supplements can play a really powerful role in improving sperm health, but only when used correctly, at the right dose, and while also addressing sleep, nutrition, regular movement, and stress management. With that foundation in place, supplements become a real game-changer rather than just another bottle on the shelf.

Now, I'll walk you through the most important and commonly used supplements for male fertility, explaining what they do, when they're useful, and what kind of impact you can realistically expect from them.

Multivitamin

It is a good foundation for covering basic nutritional needs. The problem is that not all multivitamins are created equal. Some are excellent, while others are poorly formulated, underdosed, or packed with fillers.

One important point is iron. It is essential in small amounts, but excessive amounts can cause oxidative stress, damaging sperm and testicular function. Most males have already met their iron needs through their diet, and excess iron tends to accumulate in the body rather than being excreted. This is why a multivitamin for male patients should not contain iron. Female multivitamins are different because females often lose iron through menstruation and may need more. But for males, added iron is, in most cases, unnecessary and potentially harmful.

Another key factor is folate. Folate is essential for DNA synthesis and repair, making it critical for sperm health. But not all forms of folate are equal. Many supplements still use synthetic folic acid, which is not efficiently converted into its active form, especially in patients with MTHFR gene variations. What you want to look out for are forms like methylfolate, 5-MTHF, or L-methylfolate. These are active forms that the body can use straight away, without relying on inefficient conversions. If a label only says, "folic acid," that's a red flag.

Ultimately, a multivitamin can be a great foundation for sperm health if chosen wisely. Look for active forms of vitamins and avoid unnecessary extras like iron.

B12 and folate

Low levels of B12 and folate have been linked to reduced testosterone and lower sperm count. Both nutrients are crucial for DNA replication, which makes them directly involved in sperm quality, from proper shape (morphology) to protecting against DNA fragmentation.

When assessing B12 and folate in my patients, the first step is usually a blood test.

Remember, there's a big difference between being "within the normal range" and being at truly optimal levels for fertility.

	Reference Range	Optimal reference range for fertility
Folate	7 to 40 nmol/L	> 40 nmol/L
B12	80 to 340 nmol/L	>500 nmol/L
Active B12	38 to 75 nmol/L	>100 nmol/L

Another useful way I check B12 and folate status is by looking at homocysteine in a blood test. Homocysteine is a natural byproduct of protein metabolism. Normally, your body recycles it efficiently with the help of B12, folate, and B6. But when these nutrients are low, homocysteine levels may increase.

High homocysteine can be problematic as it drives inflammation, damages blood vessels, and reduces circulation to key organs, including the testes. And when blood flow is compromised, sperm production and quality suffer. Studies have consistently shown that patients with elevated homocysteine tend to have poorer semen parameters, lower counts, reduced motility, abnormal morphology, and more DNA fragmentation.

The dosage

I usually adjust the dosage of folate and B12 for each patient depending on their homocysteine results. If you have yet to do a homocysteine test, a good place to start is around 500 mcg of activated folate and 500 mcg of activated B12 daily. Just remember that if your homocysteine is elevated, or your blood test shows low B12 or folate, you may need higher dosages to get results.

Omega-3: fish oils

Omega-3s are essential for building strong, healthy sperm. The outer layer of a sperm cell (its membrane) must be both fluid and flexible so the sperm can swim properly and reach the egg. Omega-3s are what give the membrane that strength and flexibility, which is why they're so critical for sperm motility and morphology.

But their role doesn't stop there. Omega-3s also protect sperm DNA from oxidative stress, which otherwise can increase the risk of miscarriage. They support testosterone production, keep inflammation at bay, and generally create a healthier environment for spermatogenesis.

When we talk about Omega-3s, we're mostly referring to two types: DHA and EPA. DHA plays a structural role, being a major component of the sperm cell membrane, giving it stability and flexibility. EPA, on the other hand, is involved in controlling inflammation and supporting blood flow, which is equally important for testicular and overall reproductive health. Both work hand in hand to create the conditions needed for healthy sperm development and function.

The dosage

In most cases, I recommend my patients start with 2,000mg of total Omega-3s with a combination of DHA and EPA.

Always choose supplements with 3rd-party testing for heavy metals. One of the biggest problems when it comes to Omega 3 supplementation is toxicity from heavy metals such as mercury or lead. Some companies have poor standards when it comes to purification methods and quality control.

Raul Pastrana

Vitamin D

Vitamin D isn't just important for bones and immunity; it also plays a key role in male reproductive health. It helps regulate hormone production in the testes and supports sperm development. Research shows that having too little or too much vitamin D can be linked to poorer sperm quality, including motility, concentration, and shape.

From a practical standpoint, the "sweet spot" for most men seems to be around 100 nmol/L. Levels below 50 nmol/L or above 125 nmol/L are associated with less optimal sperm parameters, while moderate levels support better overall fertility outcomes. Because everyone absorbs and responds to vitamin D differently, depending on factors like genetics, gut health, and lifestyle, the safest approach is to start with a blood test to know your baseline before supplementing.

Once you know your level, supplementation can be tailored: some patients may need very little if their levels are already adequate, while others benefit from a higher dose initially, followed by retesting to fine-tune it. This personalised approach ensures vitamin D supports fertility effectively, without risking levels that could negatively affect sperm health.

The dosage

Once you know your vitamin D level, I tailor recommendations based on where you sit:

- ☐ If your levels are close to 100 nmol/L and summer is starting where you live, you may not need any supplementation at all.

- ☐ If your levels are close to 100 nmol/L but winter is coming, a small dose of around 1,000–2,000 IU per day can help maintain healthy levels.

- ☐ If your levels are much lower than this, starting with a higher dosage can be useful. I usually recommend re-testing after 6 weeks to adjust the dose depending on how your body responds.

☐ If your levels are higher than 125 nmol/L, you don't need supplementation. In fact, it's a good idea to check any supplements you're already taking to make sure they're not adding extra vitamin D unnecessarily. Unless your doctor has told you otherwise, stopping at that point can help avoid vitamin D toxicity.

Everyone absorbs vitamin D differently. Things like gut health, body composition, and even genetics play a role, so testing is the safest way to supplement appropriately.

Lipoic acid

Alpha-lipoic acid (ALA) is a powerful antioxidant with a unique advantage as it works in both water and fat environments. That means it can protect a wide variety of cells and tissues, including sperm, from oxidative stress and damage.

There are three main situations where I find ALA especially helpful for improving sperm health:

1. **Low morphology:** When the percentage of normally shaped sperm falls below 10%, ALA can be a great addition. I usually recommend at least 3 months of supplementation.

2. **High DNA fragmentation:** If DNA fragmentation is high, antioxidants become even more important. The last two weeks of sperm development (as sperm travel through the epididymis before ejaculation) are when sperm are most vulnerable to oxidative stress. Using ALA during this window can help reduce further DNA damage and support healthier sperm DNA.

3. **Signs of poor glucose control:** In patients with insulin resistance, high insulin, or unwanted weight gain, ALA can play a dual role. Not only works by protecting sperm from oxidative stress, but it also helps stabilise blood sugar, which reduces cravings and improves appetite control. This, in turn, creates a healthier metabolic environment for sperm production.

The dosage

The typical issue is 600 to 800 mg per day, divided into 2 or 3 smaller doses. Splitting the dosage helps maintain steady levels in the body and improves its effectiveness for supporting sperm quality, protecting DNA, and assisting with glucose metabolism

Coenzyme Q10, CoQ10 or ubiquinol

CoQ10 is one of the best researched and widely accepted supplements when it comes to fertility, and for good reason. Unlike many other supplements that may target just one or two parameters, CoQ10 has been shown to improve sperm count, motility, and morphology, as well as reduce DNA fragmentation. This is due to CoQ10's central role in energy production inside the mitochondria, which are essentially the "powerhouses" of sperm cells. Since sperm need a huge amount of energy to swim all the way to the egg, better mitochondrial function often translates directly into improved sperm motility and overall function.

Another key benefit of CoQ10 is its antioxidant power. Oxidative stress is one of the most damaging factors for sperm, and CoQ10 helps protect both the sperm cell membrane and its DNA from this kind of damage. This is why I often see CoQ10 improving embryo quality in couples going through IVF.

I also always consider CoQ10 for patients taking statins. These medications (while important for managing cholesterol) lower CoQ10 levels. Replenishing those reserves not only supports sperm health but also helps with energy levels and long-term health.

Dosage

For most of my patients, the dosage I use is 300 mg per day, divided into two doses of 150 mg each. Taking CoQ10 with a meal that includes some fat improves absorption and ensures the body can use it effectively.

In cases where advanced paternal age is one of the contributing factors to poor semen results, I may increase the dosage to 600 mg per day, split into two doses of 300 mg. I only use this higher amount when I believe it's necessary, since CoQ10 can be one of the more expensive supplements, and I want my patients to get the best value out of their plan.

It's also important to know that CoQ10 comes in two forms: ubiquinone and ubiquinol. Ubiquinone is cheaper, since the body still needs to convert it into its active form before it can be used. Ubiquinol, on the other hand, is already in the active form and much easier for the body to utilise.

Raul Pastrana

NAC (n-acetyl cysteine)

NAC is a powerful antioxidant and a precursor of glutathione, which is one of the body's most important natural defences against oxidative stress. By supporting glutathione production, NAC helps to protect cells from inflammation and oxidative damage, two major factors that can compromise male fertility.

Research has shown that NAC can improve key semen parameters, including motility, concentration, and DNA fragmentation. I often recommend NAC to patients with a history of alcohol use, as it supports the liver in processing and reducing the damage caused by chronic alcohol intake. I also find it useful for patients recovering from viral infections, where oxidative stress levels tend to be higher.

That said, NAC isn't for everyone. It can thin mucus and make coughing easier, which is helpful in respiratory conditions, but in some cases, it's contraindicated. For example, individuals with active asthma may be more susceptible to bronchospasms. It may also interact with certain medications, like nitroglycerin, and is best avoided without medical supervision in those cases. It can also be challenging on the digestive system, and some people have trouble converting this precursor to glutathione and require a different approach.

Dosage

For most males, I recommend a daily dose of 1,000 to 2,000 mg, depending on the level of antioxidant support required. It's best to split this into two doses throughout the day and take it with meals to enhance absorption and minimise the risk of gastrointestinal discomfort.

Zinc

Zinc is essential for sperm production and testosterone balance. Low levels are linked to poorer sperm quality and lower testosterone, while adequate zinc supports fertility, energy, and recovery. The best way to know if you need more is through a blood test. Levels under 13 µmol/L may benefit from supplementation.

It's important to remember that more isn't always better: taking too much zinc can cause nausea, digestive upset, and interfere with other minerals like copper. Working with the right dose and form ensures your body can use zinc effectively without negative effects.

Dosage

The right zinc dosage really depends on your blood test results. I typically recommend working with doses starting around 25 mg/day and going up to 50 mg/day if needed. Always take zinc with food to reduce the risk of nausea. Some evidence also points to the benefits of irregular dosing (not daily), but this is usually best adopted after optimal levels are reached. Discuss this with your health care provider if you're not seeing the results you would expect from your zinc supplement.

The form of zinc makes a big difference. Zinc citrate is very well absorbed and is a great all-around option, while zinc picolinate tends to work best if there are gut issues or inflammation affecting absorption. These forms may be more expensive, but they're worth it because your body can use them effectively. On the other hand, cheaper forms like zinc oxide are often added by supplement companies to cut costs. Zinc oxide has very poor absorption, so it is important to note that the label may look impressive; however, your body may not actually get much benefit from it.

One thing to be mindful of is that many multivitamins already contain around 15 mg of zinc. If you're adding a separate zinc supplement on top of that, the total amount can increase quickly. That's why I always encourage retesting zinc levels after a few months of supplementation. It's the only way to know if you're in the right range, because just like being too low, having too much zinc can work against sperm health.

Raul Pastrana

Selenium

Selenium may only be needed in small amounts, but its role in male fertility is anything but small. It's essential for the proper development of sperm, particularly the tail. Without enough selenium, sperm can develop structural problems that reduce motility, making it harder for them to move efficiently and reach the egg.

I pay particular attention to selenium in patients with autoimmune conditions, thyroid dysfunction, or mercury toxicity. In these situations, selenium isn't just about sperm health. It helps regulate the immune system, protects the thyroid from inflammation and oxidative stress, and supports the body's detoxification pathways, especially in dealing with heavy metals like mercury.

The most reliable way to check your selenium status is through a plasma blood test. The usual reference range is 0.70 to 1.6 µmol/L. From my clinical experience, men who benefit from selenium support tend to do best when their levels are closer to the top end of that range, around 1.6 µmol/L, and in some cases, even higher for short periods of time (but this should always be under clinical supervision).

Dosage

The ideal dosage depends on your starting levels, but in practice, I often use 200 mcg per day for a few weeks before retesting and adjusting. Taking selenium *with* food improves absorption and ensures consistency.

It's also important to note that more is not always better. Excess selenium over long periods can become toxic. That's why testing and retesting are key to getting the benefits without the risks.

Vitamin E

Oxidative stress is one of the biggest threats to sperm quality. Because sperm membranes are packed with polyunsaturated fatty acids, they are highly sensitive to oxidative damage from reactive oxygen species (ROS). Vitamin E acts as a frontline antioxidant, helping to protect these delicate structures.

Research has shown that vitamin E can improve all major semen parameters, including count, motility, morphology, and DNA integrity. Its effects are even stronger when combined with other antioxidants such as vitamin C, selenium, and CoQ10.

One of the times I particularly like to use vitamin E is in the final two weeks before ejaculation. This is the period when sperm are travelling through the reproductive tract and are more exposed to oxidative stress. Providing extra antioxidant protection during this window can make a noticeable difference in sperm quality.

Clinically, vitamin E is particularly useful for males with poor motility or high cholesterol, since it protects both sperm membranes and improves cholesterol levels.

Dosage

A daily dose of around 1000 IU, taken with food, is usually sufficient. Because vitamin E is fat-soluble, it absorbs much better when paired with a meal.

Carnitine

Carnitine is an amino acid derivative that plays a key role in energy production, particularly in helping the mitochondria (the "power plants" of cells) burn fat for fuel. Because sperm need a huge amount of energy to swim effectively, carnitine supplementation has been proven to improve motility and overall sperm function.

Dosage

A typical therapeutic range is two to four g per day, divided into two doses. Taking it with meals improves absorption and reduces the risk of gastrointestinal discomfort (which some patients report if they take it on an empty stomach).

Arginine

Arginine is an amino acid that plays an important role in blood flow. It works by supporting the production of nitric oxide, a compound that helps relax blood vessels and improve circulation. Better circulation means more oxygen and nutrients can reach the testes, which is key for healthy sperm production. Arginine has also been shown to support erectile function, making it a valuable nutrient for males struggling with both fertility and performance issues. However, like everything, too much may contribute to oxidative stress and negatively affect sperm health. Arginine shouldn't be used by everyone as a blanket supplement for fertility, rather it's best used when there are clinical indicators of low nitric oxide.

Dosage

Clinical studies commonly range from 2 to 6 g per day, usually divided into two servings. Some people tolerate it well on an empty stomach, but if you experience mild gastrointestinal discomfort, it's perfectly fine to take it with food.

Vitamin C

Good old vitamin C. Simple, affordable, and one of my favourite supplements for male fertility. The research strongly supports its ability to boost testosterone, increase sperm count, and improve morphology. A big reason for this is its powerful antioxidant role in the testicular environment and seminal fluid, where it helps protect sperm cells from oxidative stress.

Vitamin C has also been proven to reduce DNA fragmentation, which is especially important for couples going through IVF. Better DNA integrity means better embryo quality, higher implantation rates, and a greater chance of carrying a pregnancy to term.

An occasion where I would not recommend vitamin C for fertility is in cases of iron overload. While iron is essential, too much can act like a toxin and damage sperm production and testicular function. Some patients have a genetic tendency to absorb and store excess iron, and because vitamin C increases iron absorption, it can make the problem worse. In those cases, other antioxidants are a safer choice. Because of this, I never supplement vitamin C without first understanding an individual's iron patterns and genetic tendencies.

Dosage

In clinical practice, I usually recommend between 1 and 4 grams per day, divided into 2 to 3 doses. It can be taken with or without food.

Quercetin

Quercetin is a flavonoid with strong antioxidant properties. It helps neutralise free radicals and protects sperm from oxidative stress, supporting both DNA integrity and the flexibility of the sperm membrane.

I find it especially useful for patients with varicocele. It helps strengthen blood vessel walls and promotes healthier blood flow to the testes, which is one of the key issues in varicocele-related fertility problems.

That being said, it's not suitable for everyone. At higher dosages, Quercetin can push testosterone conversion into oestrogen, which is exactly what we want to avoid if you're already dealing with low testosterone and high oestrogen levels. In those cases, I tend to avoid it or look for alternative antioxidants.

Dosage

The most common dosage range I use is 500 to 1000 mg per day, divided into two doses. Taking it with meals helps improve absorption and reduces the chance of stomach irritation.

A final note about supplementation

I've shared a lot of information on different supplements, but that doesn't mean every patient should take all of them. My role as a clinician is to look at each individual as a whole, unique strengths, weaknesses, and the specific barriers that may be affecting sperm production.

This is why I always start with the basics: blood tests, semen analysis, and a good conversation about lifestyle, stress, sleep, and nutrition. With that full picture, I can recommend the right supplements, at the best dosage, for the appropriate amount of time.

I know it can feel overwhelming. The supplement market has exploded in the last couple of decades, with countless brands making big promises. It is not always easy to know which products are high quality, which dosages are effective, and which ones are just clever marketing. I hope that this chapter has brought you some clarity about what may be most suitable for your needs. But honestly, it's only with degree qualifications in nutrition and supplementation that we really have the skills required to navigate this complex field. If you are still unsure, working with a qualified health professional who understands both male fertility and supplementation can help you make smart, targeted choices rather than guessing.

Chapter 15

Thank you

Writing this book has been both a challenge and a joy. When the idea first came to me, I wasn't sure where it would lead. Would it be an article, a short guide, or a full book? All I knew was that I had an important message to share. The thought came to me during a walk with a dear friend, and the very next morning, I began writing.

Of course, I also felt nervous. English is not my first language, so taking on a project like this meant stepping outside my comfort zone. But I decided to push through anyway.

I hope you have enjoyed reading it as much as I have enjoyed writing it, and I hope that this book has given you a deeper understanding of the importance of equal participation in fertility. Females should not carry most of the responsibility when there is a fertility challenge. Both partners matter, and both have an important role to play.

So, if you need to book a blood test, do it. If you need to make that appointment with your doctor, do it. Follow through with the necessary changes to improve the quality of your sperm, because as we have discussed repeatedly, it truly matters.

By sharing responsibility, you ease the burden your partner may have been carrying alone. That shift toward seeing fertility as fifty-fifty creates stronger couples, healthier pregnancies, and better long-term outcomes for your child. This book is my way of sharing what I've learned through years of practice, study, and supporting couples on their fertility journey. I've witnessed incredible transformations, and I know that meaningful change is possible for you too.

Remember, you do not need to do everything at once. Start with one or two areas to build momentum, and keep going. This is not only about fertility, but also about your long-term health, your energy, your confidence, and the future of your family. Finally, I would like to give a special thank you to my mentor and dear friend, Rhiannon Hardingham. Over the past four years, she has become a constant source of knowledge and inspiration. Thank you for believing in me.

<u>Let's work together</u>

If you've read this book, you already understand something most people don't:

Male fertility matters

And more importantly, it is measurable, testable, and often improvable when approached properly.

In clinic, I work with males, females and couples who want clarity, structure, and a targeted plan based on real data, not guesswork.

This often includes:

- Abnormal semen parameters
- High DNA fragmentation
- Recurrent miscarriage
- IVF preparation
- "Unexplained" infertility
- Hormonal imbalances
- Sperm and egg optimisation

My approach is structured and testing-driven. We look at what is actually happening: hormones, oxidative stress, nutrient status, metabolic markers, inflammation, gut health and environmental exposures, and build a precise plan around that.

No generic supplement protocols.

No blanket advice.

No unnecessary extremes.

If you're ready to move from information to implementation, you can book a consultation through my website:

www.rhreproductivehealth.com

I look forward to working with you.

Raul Pastrama

www.ingramcontent.com/pod-product-compliance
Lightning Source LLC
Chambersburg PA
CBHW050002040726
47599CB00014B/1183